THE CLASSIFICATION OF CHILD AND ADOLESCENT MENTAL HEALTH IN PRIMARY CARE

Diagnostic and Statistical Manual for Primary Care (DSM-PC) Child and Adolescent Version

Mark L. Wolraich, MD, Editor
Marianne E. Felice, MD, Assistant Editor
Dennis Drotar, PhD, Assistant Editor

American Academy of Pediatrics
PO Box 927
141 Northwest Point Blvd
Elk Grove Village, IL 60009-0927

Library of Congress Catalog Card No. 95-075817

ISBN No. 0-910761-71-X

MA0087

Prices on request. Address all inquiries to:
American Academy of Pediatrics, PO Box 927, 141 Northwest Point Blvd, Elk Grove Village, IL
60009-0927.

The recommendations in this publication do not indicate an exclusive course of treatment or serve as a standard of medical care. Variations, taking into account individual circumstances, may be appropriate.

Printed in the United States of America.

Task Force on Coding for Mental Health in Children

Members

Mark L. Wolraich, MD, *Chair*
Patrick Casey, MD
Marianne E. Felice, MD
Michael S. Jellinek, MD
Kelly Kelleher, MD
Judith S. Palfrey, MD
James M. Perrin, MD
Peter Rappo, MD
Esther H. Wender, MD

Liaison Representatives

Dennis Drotar, PhD,
   Society for Pediatric Psychology and Section on Clinical Child Psychology
   (American Psychological Association)
Dean H. Griffin, MD,
   American Academy of Family Physicians
Michael E. Fishman, MD,
   Health Resources and Services Administration, Maternal and Child Health Bureau
Stanley I. Greenspan, MD,
   Zero to Three/National Center for Clinical Infant Programs
Katerina Haka-Ikse, MD,
   Canadian Paediatric Society
Michael S. Jellinek, MD,
   American Academy of Child and Adolescent Psychiatry
Kathryn Magruder, PhD, MPH,
   National Institute of Mental Health
James M. Perrin, MD,
   Society for Behavioral Pediatrics
Harold Pincus, MD,
   American Psychiatric Association
Marshall Rosman, PhD,
   American Medical Association†
Serena Wieder, PhD,
   Zero to Three/National Center for Clinical Infant Programs
Consultant: Jeffrey Newcorn, MD,
      American Psychiatric Association

Staff

Jill Patterson-Mallin, MA, Project Manager
Pamela A. Rehm, MS, Program Specialist

†Deceased

CONTRIBUTORS AND CONSULTANTS

Environmental and Interactional Factors Work Group

Patrick Casey, MD, *Chair*, Little Rock, AR
Dennis Drotar, PhD, Cleveland, OH
Victor Fornari, MD, Manhasset, NY
Barbara Jo Howard, MD, Chapel Hill, NC
Jeffrey Newcorn, MD, New York, NY
Greg Prazar, MD, Exeter, NH
J. Kenneth Whitt, PhD, Chapel Hill, NC

Responses to Physical Conditions Work Group

James M. Perrin, MD, *Chair*, Boston, MA
Barbara W. Desguin, MD, Chicago, IL
Avrum L. Katcher, MD, Flemington, NJ
David Herzog, MD, Boston, MA
Gerald Koocher, PhD, Boston, MA
William MacLean, PhD, Nashville, TN
Brian McConville, MD, Cincinnati, OH†

Emotions and Moods Work Group

Kelly Kelleher, MD, *Chair*, Pittsburgh, PA
John Jemerin, MD, San Francisco, CA
Barbara Melamed, PhD, Bronx, NY
Sheridan Phillips, PhD, Baltimore, MD
Martin T. Stein, MD, LaJolla, CA
Sam Yancy, MD, Durham, NC
Consultants: Emily Harris Canning, MD, Pittsburgh, PA
Karen Rhea, MD, Nashville, TN

Disruptive Behaviors Work Group

Esther H. Wender, MD, *Chair*, Hawthorne, NY
Barry Garfinkel, MD, Minneapolis, MN
Lilly Hechtman, MD, Montreal, Quebec
Stephen Hinshaw, PhD, Berkeley, CA
Arthur Robin, PhD, Detroit, MI
Bennett A. Shaywitz, MD, New Haven, CT

Somatic Psychic Interface Work Group

Peter Rappo, MD, *Chair*, North Easton, MA
John Campo, MD, Pittsburgh, PA
Gregory Fritz, MD, Providence, RI
Judy Garber, PhD, Nashville, TN
Karen N. Olness, MD, Cleveland, OH
Neil L. Schechter, MD, Hartford, CT
C. Eugene Walker, PhD, Oklahoma City, OK
Consultants: Ron Dahl, MD, Pittsburgh, PA
             Dan Kohen, MD, Minneapolis, MN
             Mark Mahowald, MD, Minneapolis, MN
             Gerald Rosen, MD, Minneapolis, MN
             Kenneth J. Zucker, PhD, Toronto, Ontario

Cognitive and Perceptual Problems Work Group

Judith S. Palfrey, MD, *Chair*, Boston, MA
F. Curt Bennett, MD, Seattle, WA
Joel Bregman, MD, Atlanta, GA
Alberto I. Kriger, MD, Pembroke Pines, FL
Donald Routh, PhD, Coral Gables, FL
Travis Thompson, PhD, Nashville, TN
Fred Volkmar, MD, New Haven, CT
Consultant: Sally Shaywitz, MD, New Haven, CT

Severity and Functional Assessment Work Group

Michael S. Jellinek, MD, *Chair*, Boston, MA
Hector Bird, MD, New York, NY
Elizabeth Jane Costello, PhD, Durham, NC
Morris Green, MD, Indianapolis, IN
Robert Haggarty, MD, Canadaigua, NY
Woodie Kessel, MD, Rockville, MD
Julius B. Richmond, MD, Boston, MA

Formatting and Organization Work Group

Marianne E. Felice, MD, *Chair*, Baltimore, MD
Dennis Drotar, PhD, Cleveland, OH
Michael S. Jellinek, MD, Boston, MA
Peter Rappo, MD, North Easton, MA
Esther H. Wender, MD, Hawthorne, NY

Funding Sources

The development of the *DSM-PC Child and Adolescent Version* was made possible by the generous support of:

>   AAP Friends of Children Corporate Fund
>   Health Resources and Services Administration, Maternal and Child Health Bureau
>   Robert Wood Johnson Foundation

Appreciation to:

Natalie Arndt, Word Processor, Department of Maternal, Child, and Adolescent Health, American Academy of Pediatrics

Barb Scotese, Senior Medical Copy Editor, Department of Maternal, Child, and Adolescent Health, American Academy of Pediatrics

Diagnostic Classification Task Force of Zero to Three/National Center for Clinical Infant Programs and *Diagnostic Classification of Mental Health and Developmental Disorders of Infancy and Early Childhood* (DC:0-3) (Zero to Three, 1994)

TABLE OF CONTENTS

CHILD MANIFESTATIONS SECTION

DIAGNOSIS LIST

Diagnosis	Page Number	Code Number
Acculturation	48	V62.4
Acute Health Conditions	53	V61.49
Acute Stress Disorder	151	308.3
Addition of a Sibling	47	V61.8
Adjustment Disorder	312	309.xx
Adjustment Disorder With Anxious Mood	312	309.24
Adjustment Disorder With Depressed Mood	158	309.0
Adjustment Disorder With Disturbance of Conduct	130, 124	309.3
Adolescent Gender Identity Disorder	259	302.85
Adoption	45	V62.81
Adverse Effect of Work Environment	49	V62.1
Aggressive/Oppositional Problem	122	V71.02
Aggressive/Oppositional Variation	121	V65.49
Anorexia Nervosa	231	307.1
Antisocial Personality Disorder	313	301.7
Anxiety Disorder Due to a General Medical Condition	314	293.84
Anxiety Disorder, Not Otherwise Specified	163, 314	300.00
Anxiety Problem	148	V40.2
Anxiety Variation	147	V65.49
Asperger's Disorder	315	299.80
Attention-Deficit/Hyperactivity Disorder, Combined Type	98, 108	314.01
Attention-Deficit/Hyperactivity Disorder, Predominantly Hyperactive-Impulsive Type	97	314.01
Attention-Deficit/Hyperactivity Disorder, Predominantly Inattentive Type	107	314.00
Attention-Deficit/Hyperactivity Disorder, Not Otherwise Specified	98, 108	314.9
Autistic Disorder	281	299.00
Avoidant Personality Disorder	317	301.82
Bereavement	155	V62.82
Bipolar I Disorder, With Single Manic Episode	159	296.0x

Diagnosis	Page Number	Code Number
Bipolar II Disorder, Recurrent Major Depressive Episodes With Hypomanic Episodes	159	296.89
Body Dysmorphic Disorder	320	300.7
Borderline Personality Disorder	320	301.83
Breathing Related Sleep Disorder	320	780.59
Bulimia Nervosa	224	307.51
Challenges to Primary Support Group	43	V61.20
Challenges to Attachment Relationship	43	V61.20
Changes in Caregiving	45	V61.20
Change in Parental Caregiver	48	V61.0
Childhood Disintegrative Disorder	321	299.10
Childhood Gender Identity Disorder	259	302.6
Chronic Health Conditions	52	V61.49
Chronic Motor or Vocal Tic Disorder	273	307.22
Circadian Rhythm Sleep Disorder	196, 186	307.45
Communication Disorder, Not Otherwise Specified	87	307.9
Community/Social Challenges	48	V62.4
Conduct Disorder Adolescent Onset	124, 130	312.82
Conduct Disorder Childhood Onset	124, 130	312.81
Conversion Disorder	178	300.11
Cross-Gender Behavior Problem	258	V40.3
Cross-Gender Behavior Variation	257	V65.49
Cyclothymic Disorder	324	301.13
Day or Nighttime Wetting Variation	217	V65.49
Death of a Parent or Other Family Member	43	V62.82
Delirium Due to a General Medical Condition	287	293.0
Depressive Disorder, Not Otherwise Specified	158	311
Developmental/Cognitive Problem	64	V62.3
Developmental/Cognitive Variation	63	V65.49
Developmental Coordination Disorder	80	315.4
Developmental Coordination Problem	79	781.3
Developmental Coordination Variation	78	V65.49

Diagnosis	Page Number	Code Number
Dieting/Body Image Problem	230	V69.1
Dieting/Body Image Variation	229	V65.49
Discord With Peers/Teachers	49	V62.3
Dislocation	50	V60.8
Disorder of Written Expression	73	315.2
Disruptive Behaviors, Not Otherwise Specified	124, 130	312.9
Divorce	44	V61.0
Domestic Violence	44	V61.8
Dyssomnia, Not Otherwise Specified	196, 186	307.47
Dysthymic Disorder	158	300.4
Eating Disorder, Not Otherwise Specified	224, 231	307.50
Economic Challenges	51	V60.2
Educational Challenges	48	V62.3
Encopresis, With Constipation and Overflow Incontinence	212	787.6
Encopresis, Without Constipation and Overflow Incontinence	212	307.7
Enuresis	218	307.6
Excessive Nutrition Intake Problem	239	V40.3
Excessive Nutrition Intake Variation	237	V65.49
Excessive Sleepiness Problem	185	V40.3
Excessive Sleepiness Variation	184	V65.49
Expressive Language Disorder	87	315.31
Factitious Disorder	178	300.16
Factitious Disorder, Not Otherwise Specified	178	300.19
Feeding Disorder of Infancy or Early Childhood	240	307.59
Foster Care/Adoption/Institutional Care	45	V61.29
Gender Identity Disorder (Childhood Onset)	259	302.6
Gender Identity Disorder (Adolescent Onset)	259	302.85
Generalized Anxiety Disorder	149	300.02
Health-Related Behaviors Problems	250	V40.3
Health-Related Behaviors Variation	249	V65.49
Health-Related Situations	52	V61.4

Diagnosis	Page Number	Code Number
Homelessness	50	V60.0
Housing Challenges	50	V60.0
Hyperactive/Impulsive Behavior Problem	96	V40.3
Hyperactive/Impulsive Variation	95	V65.49
Hypochondriasis	330	300.7
Illiteracy of Parent	48	V62.3
Inadequate Access to Health and/or Mental Health Services	51	V61.9
Inadequate Financial Status	51	V60.2
Inadequate Housing	50	V60.1
Inadequate Nutrition Intake Problem	238	V40.3
Inadequate Nutrition Intake Variation	237	V65.4
Inadequate School Facilities	48	V62.3
Inattention Problem	106	V40.3
Inattention Variation	105	V65.49
Insomnia/Sleeplessness Problem	194	V40.3
Insomnia/Sleeplessness Variation	191	V65.49
Learning Disorder, Not Otherwise Specified	74	315.9
Learning Problem	72	V40.0
Learning Variation	71	V65.49
Legal System or Crime Problem	51	V62.5
Loss of Job	49	V62.0
Major Depressive Disorder	157	296.2x, 296.3x
Major Depressive Disorder, Single Episode	332	296.3x, 296.5x
Major Depressive Disorder, Recurrent	332	296.3x
Major Depressive Episode	331	
Marital Discord	44	V61.1
Mathematics Disorder	73	315.1
Mental Disorder of Parent	46	V61.8
Mental or Behavioral Disorder of Sibling	47	V61.8

Diagnosis	Page Number	Code Number
Mental Retardation	65	317, 318.x, 319
Mixed Receptive-Expressive Language Disorder	87	315.32
Narcolepsy	186	347
Natural Disaster	52	V62.8
Negative Emotional Behavior Problem	116	V71.02
Negative Emotional Behavior Variation	115	V65.49
Neglect	46	995.52
Nightmare Disorder	333	307.47
Nocturnal Arousals Problem	202	V40.3
Nocturnal Arousals Variation	201	V65.49
Obsessive-Compulsive Disorder	163	300.3
Oppositional Aggressive Problem	122	V71.02
Oppositional Aggressive Variation	121	V65.4
Oppositional Defiant Disorder	123	313.81
Other Environmental Situations	52	V62.8
Other Family Relationship Problems	45	V61.9
Other Functional Change in Family	47	V61.20
Pain Disorder	177	307.80
Panic Disorder	150	300.01
Panic Disorder With Agoraphobia	150	300.21
Panic Disorder Without Agoraphobia	150	300.01
Parasomnia, Not Otherwise Specified	204	307.47
Parent-Child Separation	45	V61.20
Parent or Adolescent Occupational Challenges	49	V62.2
Partial Arousals Problem	194	V40.3
Phonological Disorder	88	315.39
Physical Abuse	45	995.54
Physical Illness of Parent	47	V61.4
Physical Illness of Sibling	47	V61.4
Pica	338	307.52
Posttraumatic Stress Disorder	151	309.81

Diagnosis	Page Number	Code Number
Poverty	51	V60.2
Primary Hypersomnia	186	307.44
Primary Insomnia	196	307.42
Psychological Factors Affecting Medical Condition	251	316
Purging/Binge-Eating Problem	223	V69.1
Purging/Binge-Eating Variation	223	V65.49
Quality of Nurture Problem	46	V61.20
Reading Disorder	73	315.00
Religious or Spiritual Problem	48	V62.89
Repetitive Behaviors Problem	272	V40.3
Repetitive Behaviors Variation	271	V65.49
Rett's Disorder	341	299.80
Ritual, Obsessive, Compulsive Problem	162	V40.3
Ritual Variation	162	V65.49
Rumination Disorder	341	307.53
Sadness Problem	156	V40.3
Sadness Variation	155	V65.49
Secretive Antisocial Behaviors Problem	129	V71.02
Secretive Antisocial Behaviors Variation	129	V65.49
Separation Anxiety Disorder	150	309.21
Sexual Abuse	45	995.53
Sexual Behaviors Problem	264	V40.3
Sexual Behaviors Variation	263	V65.49
Sexual Disorder, Not Otherwise Specified	265	302.9
Sleep Terror Disorder	204	307.46
Sleeplessness Problem	194	V40.3
Sleeplessness Variation	191	V65.49
Sleepwalking Disorder	204	307.46
Social Discrimination and/or Family Isolation	48	V62.81
Social Interaction Variation	279	V65.49
Social Phobia	149	300.23
Social Withdrawal Problem	280	V40.3

Diagnosis	Page Number	Code Number
Soiling Problem	211	V40.3
Soiling Variation	211	V65.49
Somatic Complaints Problem	176	V40.3
Somatic Complaints Variation	175	V65.49
Somatoform Disorder	177	300.82
Somatoform Disorder, Not Otherwise Specified	178	300.82
Specific Phobia	149	300.29
Speech and Language Problem	86	V40.1
Speech and Language Variation	84	V65.49
Stereotypic Movement Disorder	273	307.3
Stuttering	88	307.0
Substance Abuse Disorder	139	305.xx
Substance Abusing Parents	45	V61.8
Substance Dependence	348	303.xx, 304.xx
Substance Intoxication	139	305.xx
Substance Use Problem	138	V71.09
Substance Use Variation	137	V65.49
Substance Withdrawal	139	292.0
Suicidal Ideation Problem	167	V40.2
Suicidal Ideation and Attempts	168	313.89
Thoughts of Death Problem	167	V40.2
Thoughts of Death Variation	167	V65.49
Tourette's Disorder	273	307.23
Transient Tic Disorder	273	307.21
Trichotillomania	273	312.39
Undifferentiated Somatoform Disorder	177	300.82
Unemployment	49	V62.0
Unsafe Neighborhood	50	V60.8
Witness of Violence	52	V62.89
Wetting Problem	217	V40.3
Wetting Variation	217	V65.49

Introduction

Mark L. Wolraich, MD

Purpose

The *DSM-PC Child and Adolescent Version* is intended to help primary care clinicians better identify psychosocial factors affecting their patients so that they can provide interventions when appropriate, be reimbursed for those interventions, and identify and refer patients who require more sophisticated mental health care. It is hoped that its use will stimulate further research so that subsequent revisions of the system will improve our knowledge of the range of mental health problems that occur in children and adolescents.

Primary care clinicians provide a critical point of access for children in need of mental health services. In the United States, pediatricians and family practitioners account for approximately three quarters of all office-based visits for child health care per year. In addition, these clinicians provide the vast majority of hospital-based care for children and adolescents. As such, they are the health professionals who are most likely to come in contact with children and adolescents who have behavioral and emotional problems. For primary care clinicians to address these problems, they need to be able to accurately describe and classify the phenomena they observe. For mental health clinicians the *Diagnostic and Statistical Manual of Mental Disorders,* now in its fourth revision *(DSM-IV),* and other mental health classification systems have provided this function. These systems facilitate communication among and between mental health care clinicians, health insurance agencies, and mental health researchers.

Available mental health classification systems are not widely used in primary care settings because their focus has been on the more severe and extensive conditions seen by mental health clinicians. Primary care clinicians, however, usually need to address a wide range of problematic psychosocial issues. These can include adverse psychological situations or symptoms in their patients that do not meet the criteria for a specific mental disorder and yet do require intervention. For this reason, primary care providers require a system that helps them describe these phenomena. In addition, primary care clinicians need to be able to identify and refer patients who exhibit more serious mental disorders to mental health clinicians. In such cases, primary care clinicians need to recognize these cases rather than give an exact diagnosis. Currently, the mental health classification systems provide extensive detail about mental disorders but too little detail about common problems and situations that primary care clinicians need to handle.

To address the mental health classification needs of primary care clinicians, the American Academy of Pediatrics (AAP) and American Psychiatric Association (APA) have worked collaboratively in this project to improve the classification, recognition, and diagnosis of childhood mental disorders in primary care. This parallels a collaborative project between the APA and primary care organizations that developed the *DSM-IV Primary Care Version (DSM-IV-PC).* The child and adolescent version reflects the active participation of pediatricians, child psychiatrists, and child psychologists with liaisons from the American Academy of Child and Adolescent Psychiatry, Society for Pediatric Psychology, and Section on Clinical Child Psychology of the American Psychological Association, American Academy of Family Physicians, Society for Behavioral Pediatrics, American Medical Association, Health Resources and Services Administration/ Maternal and Child Health Bureau, and National Institute of Mental Health. Representatives from the participating organizations agreed to be acknowledged as collaborators. However, the organizations were not asked to approve the document formally or review it for accuracy.

KEY ASSUMPTIONS

The *DSM-PC Child and Adolescent Version* is based on four major assumptions:

- ◆ The environments of children have an important impact on their mental health.

- ◆ A functional mental health classification system must be clear, concise, based on objective information when possible, and organized so that it can be revised and refined by subsequent research.

- ◆ In most situations, the symptoms children demonstrate vary along a continuum from normal variations to problems to disorders.

- ◆ For a mental health classification system to be useful for clinical, training, and research purposes, it must be compatible with existing systems.

ORGANIZATION OF THE MANUAL

Situations

On the basis of the first assumption, this manual is divided into two major sections. **The first section addresses the issue of a child's environment.** The *preamble* to this section is provided to help the clinician describe and consider the impact of *situations* that present in practice and affect a child's mental health. It also will help the clinician determine the potential consequences of an adverse situation and identify factors that may make the child more vulnerable or resilient and thus lessen or heighten the situation's effect. The preamble is followed by *a list of potentially adverse situations grouped by the nature of the situations* with those situations that are most common and/or well-researched more specifically defined in that section.

To help clinicians evaluate the impact of stressors, information concerning key *risk* and *protective factors* is provided in the preamble (Table 1, p 36) and under the definitions of specific stressors. In some clinical situations it may be important to identify and intervene in a stressful circumstance in order to prevent or limit adverse effects on the child. In others, it will be necessary to determine how a stressful situation affects the child's behavior. To help clinicians assess the effects of situations on children's behavior, Table 2 summarizes *common behavioral responses* to stressful events for children of various ages. Cross-referencing is also provided to guide the clinician to the relevant portion of the *child manifestation section.*

Child Manifestations

The second major section describes *child manifestations that are organized into behavioral clusters.* This format, centered on presenting symptoms, was selected because it is the most practical to use. In most cases, clinicians are first presented with concerns raised by children or their parents. By using the *index of presenting complaints* (Appendix A), clinicians can access the system based on these concerns. The clusters are also presented in an algorithmic format to facil- itate the clinician's ability to make a differential diagnosis. The format for the behavioral clusters is provided in Fig 1.

As shown in Figs 2 and 3, the design of each cluster in this section was developed to help the primary care clinician evaluate the following: 1) the spectrum of the child's symptoms, 2) common developmental presentations, and 3) the differential diagnosis. *Specific definitions or diagnostic criteria are presented in the left-hand column, and developmental presentations and special information are presented in the right-hand column.*

Spectrum Section

This classification system is based on the assumption that most behavioral manifestations reflect a spectrum from normal to disordered behavior. Accordingly, each cluster has three categories: *developmental variations, problems,* and *disorders.*

- ◆ The *developmental variations* are behaviors that parents may raise as a concern with their primary care clinician, but that are within the range of expected behaviors for the age of the child. These are most likely addressed by reassuring the parents that these are appropriate behaviors. The code provided for this, V65.49, is a nonspecific *ICD-9-CM* counseling code. We are requesting a modifier so the code will be specifically for counseling about develop- mental variation.

- ◆ The *problems* reflect behavioral manifestations that are serious enough to disrupt the child's functioning with peers, in school, and/or in the family but do not involve a sufficient level of severity/impairment to warrant the diagnosis of a mental disorder. In many cases, these may be treated with short-term counseling frequently provided by the primary care clinician. However, some of these problems will be referred to mental health practitioners for assess- ment and intervention. Otherwise, a general *ICD-9-CM* problem code is utilized.

◆ The *disorders* are those defined in *DSM-IV.* Each has specific criteria. In most cases, their presence will warrant referral to mental health clinicians. However, some disorders, such as attention-deficit/hyperactivity disorder or enuresis, have frequently been managed in primary care settings, sometimes in collaboration with mental health practitioners. For those commonly treated conditions, detailed *DSM-IV* criteria are provided in the cluster. For the other disorders, symptoms are summarized in the clusters to provide the clinician with enough information to identify the disorder. Specific detailed criteria are provided in the appendix. All disorder codes are *DSM-IV* codes. For some clusters there is a disorder condition referred to as Not Otherwise Specified (NOS); this is used if the clinical presentation conforms to the general guidelines of the disorder but does not meet all the symptom criteria, conforms to a symptom pattern not included in the *DSM-IV,* or there is insufficient opportunity to complete data collection. Use an NOS code when the condition causes clinically significant distress or impairment in most cases warranting referral to mental health clinicians. When the specific disorder criteria are not met, clinical judgment must be used to decide whether the degree of distress or impairment is mild enough to be considered a problem or severe enough to be considered an NOS disorder.

Common Developmental Presentations

The second important function of this section is to provide the clinician with developmental guidelines for coding. *This is provided in the upper right-hand box for each of the variations, problems, and disorders.* Four age periods are defined: infancy (birth to 2 years of age), early childhood (3 to 5 years of age), middle childhood (6 to 12 years of age), and adolescence (13 years of age or older). Information is provided only where the symptomatology is different for the age groups. It is also important to note that the symptoms presented are meant to be common examples, not a complete list. The developmental symptoms are presented to help the clinician recognize the expression of a problem or a disorder in different age groups. *The special information box in the lower right-hand corner provides pertinent clinical information and cross-references to situations or other problems or disorders that should be considered.*

Differential Diagnosis

The third aspect of the clusters is designed to help the primary care clinician make a differential diagnosis. The differential diagnosis issues are primarily of concern when considering the possibilities of a disorder, although some consideration should be given at the problem level. This follows the spectrum component and is divided into two sections, *alternative causes* and *comorbid and associated conditions.* The differential diagnosis component begins with those phenomena that could be alternative causes for the behaviors and is divided into three parts. The first part, in the left-hand column, lists those *general medical conditions* that could cause the child's behavioral manifestations. The list gives the most common examples and is not meant to be exhaustive. *The right-hand column labeled "special information" presents pertinent information and coding instructions.* The second part presents *substances, legal and illegal,* that may cause the behavioral manifestations. Again, the list is not meant to be all-inclusive, and pertinent information and coding instructions are provided in the right-hand column. The third part consists of *other mental disorders* that may present with similar behavioral symptoms and that, if present, should be coded in place of the disorder in the cluster.

The *comorbid section* is organized similarly to the alternative causes section with only two parts, *other mental disorders* and *general medical conditions.* However, in this case the conditions are not meant to replace the problem or disorder identified in the cluster, but may be present in addition to the other diagnosis. These are all conditions that more frequently occur simultaneously with the condition identified and should be considered. Again, these lists contain the most commonly occurring conditions that occur simultaneously and are not all-inclusive. As with the previous section, pertinent information and coding instructions are provided in the right-hand column.

With both sections of the manual, numerous *cross-references* are provided to ensure that the clinician considers *both situations* and *manifestations* for each of their patients. In many cases, both are likely to require coding. In the manifestations section the cross-references are most prominently found in the right-hand column, *Special Information.*

Severity

In order to determine needs for intervention, it is helpful to evaluate the overall severity of the child's behavioral problem and environmental situation. Severity is addressed to some extent in the spectrum section of the child manifestations because the decision about behavioral symptoms reflecting variation, problem, or disorder is a severity judgment. In addition, this manual provides clinicians with general guidelines they can use to characterize their patient's overall functioning (see *Considering the Severity of Clinical Need,* p 23). The section describes the elements that should help determine the severity of a child's condition — *symptoms, functioning, burden of suffering,* and *risk/protective factors* — and suggests using the three categories of *mild, moderate,* or *severe* to describe the severity.

Fig 1. Format for behavioral clusters.

Cluster Title

> **Presenting Complaints**

Definitions and Symptoms

Epidemiology

Etiology

Fig 2. Format for spectrum section and developmental presentations.

DEVELOPMENTAL VARIATION	COMMON DEVELOPMENTAL PRESENTATIONS
	Infancy **Early Childhood** **Middle Childhood** **Adolescence**
	SPECIAL INFORMATION

PROBLEM	COMMON DEVELOPMENTAL PRESENTATIONS
	Infancy **Early Childhood** **Middle Childhood** **Adolescence**
	SPECIAL INFORMATION

DISORDER	COMMON DEVELOPMENTAL PRESENTATIONS
	Infancy **Early Childhood** **Middle Childhood** **Adolescence**
	SPECIAL INFORMATION

Fig 3. Differential diagnosis.

DIFFERENTIAL DIAGNOSIS	SPECIAL INFORMATION
General Medical Conditions — **Examples include**	
Substances — **Examples include**	
Mental Disorders	

COMMONLY COMORBID CONDITIONS	SPECIAL INFORMATION
Other Comorbid Mental Health Conditions — Examples include	
Other General Medical Conditions — Examples include	

USING THE MANUAL

Locating Information That You Need

This manual is organized to provide easy access to the classification system by multiple methods. Consequently, practitioners should familiarize themselves with the diagnosis list, presenting complaints appendix, and child manifestation and situation list and carefully read the section on the organization of the manual. Key information is located as follows:

For those who require only the name and code number for a particular condition or situation, the *Diagnosis List* at the beginning of the manual provides this information, where the name, code number, and page numbers of the conditions can be found.

For those who wish to address a presenting complaint, an appendix of *Presenting Complaints* is provided. The presenting complaints are only pertinent to child manifestations. This index will direct the clinician to the appropriate behavioral clusters in the *Child Manifestations Section*. Those having situation-presenting complaints should consult the *Situations Section*, Table 3, on p 39.

Those who wish to obtain a better overall understanding and approach to the evaluation and coding of psychosocial problems should read the preambles to the *Situations* and *Child Manifestations Sections* and the *Section on Severity*. For those who want to understand the spectrum of manifestations for a particular childhood manifestation, the *Table of Contents* provides listings and page numbers for each cluster.

Steps in Coding Behavioral Problems and Situations

This manual is organized to provide the clinician with diagnostic categories both for the *child's environment* (situations) and the *child's behavior* (child manifestations). In some cases, the reason for a visit may relate solely to a situational concern or child behavior. However, in most cases *both* elements should be coded. The following flow chart (Fig 4) provides a step-by-step guide for using the system.

Fig 4. Flow chart of steps in coding.

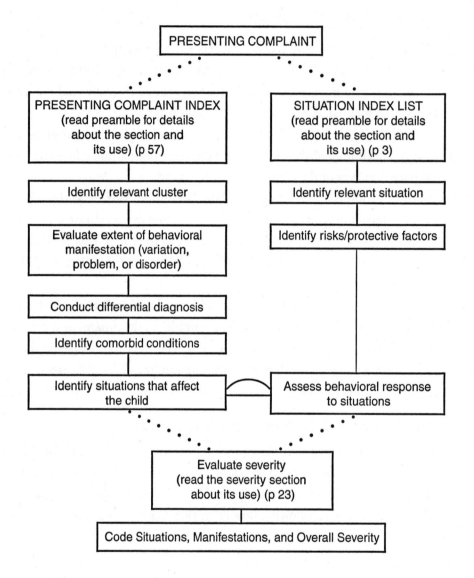

Determining the Primary Diagnosis

The *primary diagnosis is the most important focus of clinical concern.* When a developmental variation, problem, or disorder is present and is the primary focus of intervention, this should be the primary diagnosis. On the other hand, if a stressful situation is the primary focus of clinical concern, e.g., helping the child and family manage the stress of a divorce, this should be considered the primary diagnosis. Since in most situations it will not be possible to determine that a stressful situation is the exclusive direct cause of the child manifestations, both the stressor and the manifestation need to be listed. If the intent of the visit is focused on the stressor, this should be listed first. Differential diagnosis and comorbidity should be considered primarily when considering disorder diagnoses.

Case Illustrations of How To Use the Manual

Two case examples are also provided to illustrate how to use the manual.

CASE 1 — Presenting Complaints

"Interrupting class and restless (all wound up)."

History — Corey's mother tells the pediatrician that she is beginning to be concerned about the reports she receives from school that Corey, age 6, sometimes disrupts the classroom with talking out of turn and saying things that aren't related to what the class is doing. Corey's parents have been concerned about Corey since about 4 years of age because he often seems "all wound up" and is difficult to settle down for naps or at mealtimes. In addition, when asked to put away his toys or get ready for bed, he sometimes becomes resistant and has temper tantrums. Sometimes babysitters have reported that they have a hard time getting him to get ready for bed, or put away his things. Last year's kindergarten teacher reported that Corey was "high spirited" but felt he contributed to the class and was just "a little immature."

Corey is the first child of parents who both work "to make ends meet." A younger female sibling was born 2 years ago and the parents feel that Corey's problems really became apparent then. An added concern is the father's recent loss of job due to his company downsizing. The mother continues to work full-time while the father is job hunting.

The teacher reports that Corey is learning to read and does average work in math. He particularly likes music and the teacher finds that she can calm him down by playing music in the classroom.

Corey has a normal early medical history except for frequent ear infections between 18 months and 3 years of age. However, the last ear infection was a little more than 1 year ago and a hearing test then was normal.

Discussion — Corey had behavioral symptoms in the hyperactive/impulsive cluster. They have caused problems that require some intervention, but these behaviors are not sufficiently pervasive to warrant the diagnosis of ADHD. Two situations (birth of a sibling and paternal job loss) appear to be contributing to the problem, the greater one at this point being the father's job loss. Given the potential effects of these situations, clinicians should also consider the fact that the behaviors may be manifestations of anxiety or depression.

Diagnosis — Hyperactivity/Impulsive Behavior Problem (V40.3); Need to rule out Major Depressive Disorder (296.2x); Marital Discord (V61.1); Severity — Mild/Moderate.

Intervention — are likely to include counseling the parents on effective parenting techniques including the need to provide individual positive attention to Corey within the framework of their current financial and job situations, and counseling them about the impact of having an additional sibling. In terms of overall severity, it appears in the mild to low moderate range. However, Corey needs to be followed closely and reevaluated because the stressors could lead to a worsening situation and the added demands of school as he gets older may bring out more symptoms.

CASE 2 — Presenting Complaint

Denying problems.

History — Thomas, age 14, was confirmed to have cystic fibrosis at 10 weeks of age following a series of respiratory infections. He has attended a cystic fibrosis special center, but not always consistently. Despite this he has done reasonably well, but recurrent respiratory infections have resulted in mild tachypnea. He becomes distinctly short of breath with exercise. He is not a tall boy and has not entered puberty. He takes medication, but does not always adhere to recommended schedules. Caloric intake was more of a problem when he was younger; however, because he does not consistently take his pancreatic granules, digestive efficiency is less than it should be. He is passing his subjects at school, but misses an average of 8 to 10 days a year for acute illnesses. Thomas' parents are separated; he lives with his father who is employed as a salesman. His hours are irregular. As a result, Thomas is not supervised for taking his medications.

Behaviorally, Thomas appears confident to the point of cockiness. He denies having any problems. When he could not make the school team because of dyspnea on exertion, he announced that he had not really wanted to play in team sports. He always has a reason for not adhering to recommendations. He asks why he can't have medicine to "get rid" of his cystic fibrosis. In private conversation, however, he spontaneously mentions difficulty in sleeping, lack of energy, worry about what will become of him, and wonders if it is worthwhile to keep on living. His father is critical of his behavior and has stated that if Thomas would only do as he is told he would have no problems.

Discussion — The patient is showing signs of depression and possible suicidal ideation. It is important to make sure that this condition is not at a disorder level; this patient should be referred to a mental health clinician to make recommendations for intervention. The patient also is not dealing effectively with his cystic fibrosis. His presenting problem is at least at a level of a health-related behavior problem or Psychological Factors Affecting Medical Conditions (316). His father's unrealistic expectations and his parents' separation contribute to his problems. The overall severity is at least moderate but possibly severe.

Diagnosis — Need to rule out Depressive Disorder (296.2xx); Health-Related Behaviors Problem (V40.3); Chronic Health Conditions (V61.49); Thoughts of Death Problem (V40.2); Need to rule out Depressive Disorder (296); Marital Discord (V61.1); Severity — Moderate (possibly Severe).

Intervention — On the basis of the concern for the presence of the depressive disorder, the child needs further evaluation by a mental health clinician, and therapy is dependent on determining whether a depressive disorder is present. The patient may benefit from psychotherapy. In all likelihood, the parents will need guidance to help them manage their son's behavior and treatment regimen for the cystic fibrosis more effectively.

Considering the Severity of Clinical Need

A primary goal of assessing, understanding, and, if necessary, intervening on behalf of a child is to support the child's long-term development of autonomy, adaptability, self-esteem, and capacity for intimacy. Epidemiological studies report that a substantial percentage (12% to over 30% depending on the choice of sample and criteria) of children in the United States have a psychosocial problem that may impede their functioning and development. These findings are not surprising to primary care clinicians who daily encounter a wide range of significant psychosocial problems as well as parents seeking guidance regarding their children's behavior and development. A key aspect of effectively evaluating parental concerns or a child's behavior is an assessment of the severity of clinical need.

Severity is an elusive concept whether applied to an acute injury, a chronic disease, or a psychosocial disorder. The narrower and more specific the issue, the easier it is to define severity. For example, it can be commonly agreed that a limited range of motion in a joint is rated or described as being "moderate in severity." However, when a child's psychosocial difficulties in a primary care setting are considered, the rating of severity requires a much more global clinical judgment that incorporates the child's and family's overall status. Consequently, the definition of severity in this manual is not limited to the child's disorder but is a comprehensive judgment that communicates the relevant urgency and seriousness of clinical needs.

Severity has four dimensions, including *symptoms, dysfunction,* the *burden of suffering on the child and family,* and *risk and protective factors.* With sufficient time, many of these dimensions can be assessed through thoughtful clinical interviewing, many may be quantified using available research methodologies, although qualitative differences are also important. In clinical practice, however, pediatricians and family practitioners usually rely on clinical judgment both to focus gathering of data and integrate the available information to determine the need for any further actions. For example, adolescent depression may reflect a transient mood state provoked by a circumstance (peer rejection) or a serious disorder that underlies suicidal ideation, substance abuse, or life-threatening behavior. The primary care clinician must weigh all available historical, developmental, symptomatic, functional, and other relevant information (e.g., family psychiatric history) to evaluate the severity of the patient's depression.

On the basis of the combination of diagnosis and rating of severity, the primary care clinician determines if further intervention is warranted (ranging from empathic listening to urgent referral to a mental health practitioner). Thus, a careful assessment of severity helps to translate a diagnostic system into clinical realities. In emergency situations such assessment may need to take place at one visit; in less emergent situations it may reflect the clinician's detailed knowledge of the family based on an ongoing relationship and multiple contacts.

Areas of Assessment

After recognition of a psychosocial disorder, the approach to assessing severity includes four dimensions: symptoms, functioning, burden of suffering, and risks/protective factors (Table 1, p 36).

Symptoms

Symptoms (sadness, anxiety, or impulsivity) should be evaluated on the basis of frequency, intensity, seriousness, duration, site of occurrence (home, school, or both), and their relationships to the differential diagnosis. In most cases, the primary care clinician evaluates all aspects of severity, especially functional impairment. However, some symptoms may occur at a level of severity that demands immediate clinical attention. For example, suicidal ideation may be sufficiently intense and/or frequent to require immediate clinical intervention.

Functioning

Symptoms, if sufficiently intense, frequent, or of longstanding duration, are likely to result in impaired functioning in one or more areas of the child's life. This impact on the child's functioning is often the most critical parameter in assessing severity. Major areas of functioning for school-age children include school, peer relationships, family, and play activities. Of course, functioning in one area can have an impact on functioning in another (for example, poor school performance can limit athletic eligibility). Also, impaired functioning may contribute to symptoms such as dysphoric mood or, over time, the child's sense of self-esteem. The duration, extent, and pervasiveness of dysfunction determine how difficult it will be for a child to attain age-appropriate developmental progress.

Burden of Suffering

A highly subjective, but important, component of severity assesses the depth of a child's and family's distress, anguish, and difficulty coping with their problems. Children and families cope with and react differently to symptoms, dysfunction, and risk factors. Suffering is a dimension that describes the individual child's and family's internal reaction to and distress concerning their presenting problems. By adding this dimension, the primary care clinician is encouraged to understand the child's and family's reaction and the urgency of their clinical needs. The burden of suffering includes the following:

- intensity of the child's personal suffering or distress
- intrusiveness of the symptoms or dysfunction in the major areas of a child's life
- duration of suffering
- limitations on the family

- increase in family or peer conflict

- danger to self or others

- variance with normative expectations

- expected course and duration of behavioral problem

Risk/Protective Factors

The presence of risk factors increases the probability that a child will need further assessment and intervention. Clinical judgments are necessary to assess the contribution of risk factors relevant to a specific child's disorder. Research findings have not as yet established relative weights for different risk factors (e.g., poverty versus divorce or chronic illness). Each risk factor affects different families and children in different ways. However, the presence of three or more risk factors may exceed the capacity of many families and children to adapt and function well, and their impact should be carefully evaluated.

The specific techniques of risk assessment that have been developed to date were not designed for brevity or clinical settings. Therefore, identifying risk factors likely to be relevant for a specific family is probably best done through the interview.

Protective factors are just as important in assessing risk and severity as risk factors. Most of these are the polar opposite of risk factors — for example, doing well in school versus not doing well in school or having an even temperament as opposed to a difficult temperament. Just as multiple risk factors geometrically increase the likelihood of more severe psychological problems, it is likely that the presence of several protective factors balances the negative impact of risk factors. For example, a child's problem might well be considered to be less severe if there was no family history of psychiatric disease, if the child was doing well in school, and the child had an even temperament and many friends. General guidelines for considering risk and protective factors are provided in the preamble of the *Situations Section*, and specific guidelines are provided with the definitions of specific stressors (pp 31 to 56).

Rating

How should the clinician communicate the severity of a situation or child manifestation? A numerical scale that reflects severity may convey a false, unreliable, or invalid sense of precision. Other descriptive scales attempt to operationalize or put a general level of functioning into words, but these may be quite cumbersome in primary care settings. A more precise attempt to describe or rate each dimension of severity (symptoms, functional impairment, suffering, and risk/protective factors) or each specific area of dysfunction would be complex, time-consuming, and require a clinical judgment as to which are the most critical factors that will determine future actions. The primary care clinician would still have to weigh and decide the overall severity based on all available information factors. The guidelines for severity will help the clinician in considering patient status, particularly in regard to developmental variations, problems, and disorders. This suggested classification of severity is different from the *DSM-IV* categorization of disorders into mild, moderate, and severe. The guidelines for this manual do not require the rating of severity for each condition individually. This manual suggests that the clinician use the following guidelines to reflect a global rating of severity:

Mild: Unlikely to cause serious developmental difficulties or impairment of functioning.

Moderate: May cause, or is causing, some developmental difficulties or impairment. Further evaluation and intervention planning are warranted.

Severe: Is causing serious developmental difficulties and dysfunction in one or more key areas of the child's life. Mental health referral and comprehensive treatment planning are often indicated, possibly on an urgent basis.

Developmental Considerations in Assessing Severity

Infancy and Early Childhood

Infant and early childhood disorders can be obvious or quite subtle. Serious disorders such as failure to thrive or pervasive developmental disorders are more easily recognized than more subtle problems. In assessing very young children, primary care clinicians traditionally use developmental measures including growth, progress through expected milestones, and their considerable experience in assessing the young child's ability to relate. Young children are less able to describe their feelings and historical events. Thus, information from parents and other caregivers and informants such as teachers is of primary significance. Assessing areas of concern (such as maternal depression, family discord, or maltreatment) that can have a serious impact on infants and toddlers requires specialized skills and is often time consuming. Evaluating a young child often requires longer interviews, and careful assessment of the child's temperament, language skills, and ability to relate, and of the family's functioning.

School Age

Developmentally, the school child is able to discuss feelings and events directly, and is expected to be functional in a wide range of areas including family, friends, school, and activities; therefore, children should be included as a source of information in the context of data from parents and teachers. Some problems such as attention-deficit/hyperactivity disorder are more overt and easily recognized than, for example, depression, sexual abuse, or learning disorders. Once a psychosocial concern is identified by parents, school personnel, questionnaire responses, or observation, the primary care clinician often continues the assessment of severity through a brief interview.

Adolescence

Many of the issues that apply to the older school-age child are also relevant to adolescents. Developmentally, adolescents are capable of contributing to both the recognition and further assessment of their psychosocial concerns. In addition, adolescents have a more complex range of feelings, areas of functioning, activities, and relationships. They face numerous issues, including autonomy, sexuality, use of alcohol or other drugs, and a higher incidence of psychiatric disorders such as depression and psychoses. Information from the parents must be augmented by the adolescent's self-report and data from external sources such as school personnel. The adolescent's multiple areas of functioning as well as respect for the privacy of his or her personal feelings and mood state must be integrated into the overall assessment of severity.

Conclusion

Just as in evaluating other medical conditions, assessing the severity of a psychosocial problem often requires a thoughtful approach, skill, and time. In addition, much may depend on the clinician's relationship with the family, training, experience with psychosocial disorders, and attitude. Although many aspects of severity can be evaluated, no simple, one-dimensional approach adequately integrates the domains of symptoms, functioning, personal suffering, and risk/protective factors. The approach outlined in this manual is intended to serve as a conceptual framework to help the clinician consider severity in a systematic manner in order to reach clinically sound decisions. Although advances in questionnaire design, research methodology, and understanding of child development continue to bring the field closer to statistically valid and reliable measurement of severity, at this time we recommend that the primary care clinician use a systematic, thoughtful, and empathic clinical approach to assess the global severity of the child's disorder.

SITUATIONS SECTION

CHILDREN'S RESPONSES TO ENVIRONMENTAL SITUATIONS AND POTENTIALLY STRESSFUL EVENTS PREAMBLE

A critical influence on children's general well-being — including behavioral and cognitive functioning and physical health — is the quality of the environment in which the child lives. A basic tenet of this manual is the central importance of the transaction over time between the child and the environment in which the child lives and grows. Child health care providers constantly make clinical judgments, both diagnostic and therapeutic, based on positive and negative characteristics of the child, the environment, and the interaction between them. *Environmental situations and potentially stressful events* that may affect the child's behavior will be addressed in this section. More detailed instructions regarding the use of this section are also included in the introduction to the manual (see p 9).

Environment includes the immediate household and its members, as well as the extended family, neighborhood, community, and cultural context. Within this broad definition, many situations may influence children's mental health functioning, including acute stressful events, such as the witnessing of violence; chronic circumstances, such as marital discord or living in poverty; and conditions having both immediate impact and enduring effects, such as the death of a parent. Environmental situations and stressful events may be associated with but not directly related to the child's behavioral symptoms, they may *act to modify (increase or lessen)* the effects of preexisting problems or disorders, or they may be *etiologically related* to the child's symptoms, such as in the case of adjustment disorders.

Emotional and behavioral symptoms observed in children that relate to environmental situations and stressful events range from minor behavioral variations of normal development, to specific behaviors or clusters of symptoms that have the potential to become pathologic, to clear-cut emotional disorders (Table 2). Stressful environmental circumstances often seem to trigger a common set of behavioral or emotional reactions in children. Few specific symptoms or disorders are known to result directly from specific situational events. Rather, the reaction of an infant, child, or adolescent to environmental situations and stressful events reflects not only the *characteristics of the stressor* (e.g., severity and intensity ["toxicity"], chronicity, number of concurrent stressors), but also the *strengths of the child and family/environment* (protective factors) and *vulnerabilities* (risk factors) (see *Considering the Severity of Clinical Need,* p 23, and Table 1, p 36).

Clinical Utility

There are several practical reasons for identifying environmental stressors, risks, and protective factors. In some cases, they may be a primary focus of clinical attention from a preventive standpoint, providing anticipatory guidance to parents in order to help them recognize and understand their child's response to stress and providing appropriate support, may help lessen the intensity of this response. It is also useful to monitor for prolonged or intense responses to stressors that may signal a behavioral problem or disorder that will require more intensive counseling or management.

A range of strategies may be employed to manage a child's and family's response to stressful situations. For example, enhancing support for the parent and child may be the clinical strategy of choice in cases in which risk factors are either difficult to identify in advance (such as dysfunctional parenting) or to eliminate altogether (such as extreme poverty). At other times, specific behavioral and cognitive skills might be taught in order to help a child or adolescent cope with stressful situations and thus reduce the potential for developing psychological symptoms.

Environmental Situations and Potentially Stressful Events

Environmental situations that affect a child's adjustment may be overlooked unless one inquires directly about them. For this reason, identification of clinically relevant environmental context problems is an important aspect of clinical management. An *Environmental Situations and Potentially Stressful Events Checklist*, which may be used to facilitate this review, is given in Table 3. This checklist is grouped into nine categories, many with subcategories. Appropriate diagnostic codes from *ICD-9-CM* are provided in this list. Pediatric clinicians may choose to use these codes as primary or secondary diagnoses if the situation is the primary reason for the clinic visit, or if the child's manifestations are a developmental variation or problem that has resulted from the situation and for which there is no separate diagnostic code.

This list is meant to depict reasonably common situations and events, and is not intended to be a totally inclusive list. While some of the events included in this checklist would be expected to be uniformly stressful, such as parental death, others may not always result in stress, depending on the risk and protective features of the child and environment.

In addition to this listing, information regarding specific environmental situations and stressful events is presented later in *Environmental Situations Defined,* p 41. Only certain situations and events from the *Environmental Situations and Stressful Events Checklist* (Table 3) are treated in this format, either because of common occurrence, or because information regarding developmental issues, vulnerabilities, and strengths associated with the specific situation or stressful event is known.

Assessment of Risk and Protective Factors

Assessment of risk factors and protective factors that may contribute to the child's mental health behavior is very helpful when evaluating a child's response to environmental stressors. *Risk factors* are associated with vulnerability — a higher probability of onset, greater severity, and longer duration of major mental health problems. *Protective factors*, in contrast, refer to attributes or situations associated with an individual's resilience or resistance to the negative effects of stress and disorder.

Specific disorders are typically associated with multiple risk factors and stressful events, rather than a single factor or event. Likewise, a single risk factor rarely predisposes a child to a particular disorder. Some risk factors predict dysfunction mainly during specific periods of development, whereas other risks are stable predictors of disorder across the life span.

Table 1 lists some risk and protective features of children and their environments that may affect their reactions to stressful events. For example, a stressful event for a child, such as the death of a loved one, may elicit varied responses from a child depending on characteristics of his or her temperament and environment (such as the amount of emotional and physical support available to the child and family from others). The list of risk and protective factors given in Table 1 is not intended to be exhaustive or even mutually exclusive, but includes many important features that a clinician may need to consider for purposes of assessment and management. It is important that all of these features be interpreted in the context of family and regional cultures and beliefs.

The risk and protective factors are *not* provided to confirm diagnoses. Criteria for diagnoses of specific problems and disorders are provided in the individual Child Manifestation Behavioral clusters. Rather, these factors are provided for the primary care provider to consider in the diagnostic process and treatment planning, when evaluating the relationship between environmental circumstances and events to child symptoms, problems, or disorders. In addition, providers may also consider directing therapeutic interventions at these child and environmental risk factors.

The *child's health* is listed in Table 1 as a risk/protective factor that may positively or negatively affect response to a range of environmental situations and stressful events. *Acute, recurrent, and chronic physical illnesses and physical impairments* such as cerebral palsy, as well as their treatments, may also be viewed as stressful contextual situations. Physical illness and impairment have a salient impact on the psychological functioning of children and create predictable demands and burdens for their families. Although, in some instances, such challenges can have a positive effect on adaptation and personal growth, the more common effect is disruptive and may range from minor behavioral variations and problems to mental disorders.

The influence of chronic conditions on a child's development varies according to the stage of life when the condition appears. Moreover, some chronic illnesses have direct effects on a child's cognition. More commonly, the cognitive abilities of children are indirectly affected, either by medications (e.g., drugs for asthma or seizure disorders that can affect cognition), by excessive fatigue and difficulties in maintaining attention, by interruptions of education, or by social isolation. Parents and siblings also face considerable adjustment tasks when a family member has a chronic physical condition. Changes in home routines, increased family financial and treatment responsibilities, and the adjustment to a child who is different from what was expected are some common burdens (see Health-Related Situations clusters, p 52).

Child characteristics to be considered as potential risk or protective characteristics include health (good health versus ill health), temperament ("easy, adaptable" versus "difficult, unadaptable"), cognitive status (normal IQ versus below normal IQ), general developmental status (normal versus delayed), emotional health (normal mental health function versus preexisting emotional disorder), sociability (good peer relations versus poor peer relations), and the child's general reaction to stress (does not blame self versus blames self).

A child's *temperament*, his or her behavioral style, is an overriding characteristic that strongly affects how children experience and react to environmental influences. In fact, parental concerns about normal variations in temperament can often be a focus of a primary care visit and anticipatory guidance. Temperament may affect not only the child's development and behavior, but also the parent-child interaction and the parents themselves. Temperament can be clinically significant either as a factor that predisposes the child to a wide range of behavior problems, e.g., sleep and feeding disturbances, or as a source of parental concern because of the way it complicates the child's care and management.

Many characteristics of temperament are clinically relevant. These include *activity*, the amount of physical motion during sleep and play; *rhythmicity*, the regularity of physiological functions such as hunger and sleep; *approach*, the nature of the initial response to new stimuli, such as people and new situations; *adaptability*, the ease or difficulty with which reactions of stimuli can be modified in a desired way; *intensity*, the energy level of responses regardless of quality or direction; *mood*, the amount of pleasant and friendly or unpleasant and unfriendly behavior in various situations; *persistence and attention span*, the length of time particular activities are pursued by the child; *distractibility*, the degree to which extraneous stimuli interfere with ongoing behavior; and *sensory threshold*, the amount of stimulation, such as sight or sound, necessary to evoke discernible responses in the child.

The *quality and continuity of the attachment relationship and caregiving* is another critical risk or protective feature, with high-quality, continuous caregiving and secure attachment considered protective, and low-quality, discontinuous caregiving with ambivalent, insecure attachment considered a risk factor. Other environmental characteristics to be considered as potential protective or risk characteristics include family resources (adequate financial resources versus poverty), quality, stability, and safety of the physical environment (adequate, stable, safe versus inadequate, unstable, unsafe), family relationships (good communication with well-defined roles versus poor communication and poorly defined roles), emotional and physical support (high support versus low support), emotional and physical health of caregivers (caregivers in good emotional and physical health versus mental illness, physical illness in caregivers), caregiver reaction to stress (adaptive/stable versus maladaptive/disruptive), and availability and access to community resources (high access versus low access).

Common Behavioral/Developmental Reactions to Environmental Situations and Stressful Events

Specific environmental situations and stressful events rarely produce specific symptoms but generally lead to similar behavioral reactions in children. Examples of common behavioral responses that *may* result from any or all environmental situations and stressful events for infants-toddlers, for early childhood, later childhood, and for adolescence are listed in Table 2. The behavioral manifestations are listed by developmental stage under the major categories of

Developmental Competency; Impulsive/Hyperactive or Inattentive Behaviors; Negative/
Antisocial Behaviors; Substance Use/Abuse; Emotions and Moods; Somatic and Sleep Behaviors;
Feeding, Eating, Elimination Behaviors; Illness-Related Behaviors; Sexual Behaviors; and
Atypical Behaviors.

Identifying the Child's Behavioral Response to Stressful Events: Case Example

Table 2 enables the primary care physician to gain access to appropriate child behavioral manifestations in other parts of this manual. Providers should also take special note of the category
of *adjustment disorders*, which reflects the development of clinically significant behavioral or
emotional symptoms in response to psychosocial stressors. As much as possible, specific behavioral manifestations and disorders listed in Table 2 are cross-referenced to specific pages in the
child behavioral manifestations section where they are discussed in more detail.

For example, a primary care provider may be asked to see a 5-year-old child by the parent
for a checkup due to a recent unpleasant divorce. While obtaining a history, the provider learns
of a change of sleeping habit of 2 weeks' duration. By referring to Table 2, *Common Behavioral
Responses to Environmental Situations and Potentially Stressful Events*, the provider notes that
change in sleep is a common behavioral reaction for a 5-year-old. This table also references
Anxious Symptoms cluster (p 145), Sadness and Related Symptoms cluster (p 153), and the
Sleeplessness cluster (p 189).

After reviewing these clusters and the development variations, problems, and disorders
described, the provider determines the child has a Sadness Problem. The provider decides to code
Divorce (V61.0) first and Sadness Problem (V40.3) second. This case illustrates how providers
may use Table 2 as guide to manifestations and disorders discussed in the *Child* section of the
manual, even while beginning with an environmental situation.

Table 1. Risk and Protective Factors		
	Protective — Decreased Impact of Stress	**Risk — Increased Impact of Stress**
Child		
Health	Good health	Ill health, chronic or acute
Temperament (p 34)	Pleasant mood, adaptable	Unpleasant mood, unadaptable
Cognitive status	Normal IQ (particularly verbal skills and abstract reasoning)	Low IQ
Emotional health	Child's capacity for adaptation based on good mental health function	Preexisting emotional disorder
Sociability	Good peer relations	Poor peer relations
Reaction to stress	Perceives stress as limited, does not blame self	Perceives continued threat, blames self
Interaction		
Quality and continuity of attachment and caregiving	High quality, continuous, securely attached	Low quality, discontinuous, ambivalent, insecurely attached
Environment		
Parent competence	Knowledgeable, experienced, competent	Poor knowledge, inexperienced, low level of competency
Family resources	Adequate economic resources	Poverty
Quality, stability, safety of environment	Adequate, stable, safe	Inadequate, unstable, unsafe
Family relationships (communication, roles)	Good communication, little conflict	Poor communication, much conflict
Emotional and physical support	High level of support	Low level of support
Emotional and physical health of caregivers	Good emotional and physical health	Mental illness, physical illness
Caregiver reaction to stress	Adaptive, stable	Maladaptive, disruptive
Availability/access to community resources	Good access	Poor access

Table 2.

Common Behavioral Responses to Environmental Situations and Potentially Stressful Events

INFANCY-TODDLERHOOD (0-2 Y)	EARLY CHILDHOOD (3-5 Y)
BEHAVIORAL MANIFESTATIONS	***BEHAVIORAL MANIFESTATIONS***
Illness-Related Behaviors N/A	**Illness-Related Behaviors** N/A
Emotions and Moods Change in crying Change in mood Sullen, withdrawn	**Emotions and Moods** Generally sad Self-destructive behaviors
Impulsive/Hyperactive or Inattentive Behaviors Increased activity	**Impulsive/Hyperactive or Inattentive Behaviors** Inattention High activity level
Negative/Antisocial Behaviors Aversive behaviors, i.e., temper tantrum, angry outburst	**Negative/Antisocial Behaviors** Tantrums Negativism Aggression Uncontrolled, noncompliant
Feeding, Eating, Elimination Behaviors Change in eating Self-induced vomiting Nonspecific diarrhea, vomiting	**Feeding, Eating, Elimination Behaviors** Change in eating Fecal soiling Bedwetting
Somatic and Sleep Behaviors Change in sleep	**Somatic and Sleep Behaviors** Change in sleep
Developmental Competency Regression or delay in developmental attainments Inability to engage in or sustain play	**Developmental Competency** Regression or delay in developmental attainments
Sexual Behaviors Arousal behaviors	**Sexual Behaviors** Preoccupation with sexual issues
Relationship Behaviors Extreme distress with separation Absence of distress with separation Indiscriminate social interactions Excessive clinging Gaze avoidance, hypervigilant gaze	**Relationship Behaviors** Ambivalence toward independence Socially withdrawn, isolated Excessive clinging Separation fears Fear of being alone
DISORDERS THAT MAY RESULT *(see Specific Child Manifestation Clusters for* *additional information)* Depression (p 153) Feeding disorder of infancy or early childhood (p 235) Insomnia (p 189)/Hypersomnia (p 181) Adjustment disorder (p 312)	***DISORDERS THAT MAY RESULT*** *(see Specific Child Manifestation Clusters for* *additional information)* Generalized anxiety disorder (p 145) Posttraumatic stress disorder (p 145) Depression (p 153) Feeding disorder of infancy or early childhood (p 235) Insomnia (p 189)/Hypersomnia (p 181) Encopresis (p 209) Enuresis (p 215) Phobia (p 145) Adjustment disorder (p 312)

Table 2.

Common Behavioral Responses to Environmental Situations and Potentially Stressful Events

MIDDLE CHILDHOOD (6-12 Y)	ADOLESCENCE (13-21 Y)
BEHAVIORAL MANIFESTATIONS	***BEHAVIORAL MANIFESTATIONS***
Illness-Related Behaviors Transient physical complaints	**Illness-Related Behaviors** Transient physical complaints
Emotions and Moods Sadness Anxiety Changes in mood Preoccupation with stressful situations Self-destructive Fear of specific situations Decreased self-esteem	**Emotions and Moods** Sadness Self-destructive Anxiety Preoccupation with stress Decreased self-esteem Change in mood
Impulsive/Hyperactive or Inattentive Behaviors Inattention High activity level Impulsivity	**Impulsive/Hyperactive or Inattentive Behaviors** Inattention Impulsivity High activity level
Negative/Antisocial Behaviors Aggression Noncompliant Negativistic	**Negative/Antisocial Behaviors** Aggression Antisocial behavior
Feeding, Eating, Elimination Behaviors Change in eating Transient enuresis, encopresis	**Feeding, Eating, Elimination Behaviors** Change in appetite Inadequate eating habits
Somatic and Sleep Behaviors Change in sleep	**Somatic and Sleep Behaviors** Inadequate sleeping habits Oversleeping
Developmental Competency Decrease in academic performance	**Developmental Competency** Decrease in academic achievement
Sexual Behaviors Preoccupation with sexual issues	**Sexual Behaviors** Preoccupation with sexual issues
Relationship Behaviors Change in school activities Change in social interaction such as withdrawal Separation fear Fear of being alone	**Relationship Behaviors** Change in school activities School absences Change in social interaction such as withdrawal
Substance Use/Abuse	**Substance Use/Abuse**
DISORDERS THAT MAY RESULT *(see Specific Child Manifestation Clusters for additional information)* Oppositional defiant disorder (see p 119) Conduct disorder (p 119) Generalized anxiety disorder (p 145) Posttraumatic stress disorder (p 145) Adjustment disorder (p 312) Depression (p 153) Somatoform disorder (p 173) Enuresis (p 215) Encopresis (p 209) Anorexia (p 227)/Bulimia (p 221) Insomnia (p 189)/Hypersomnia (p 181) Phobia (p 145)	***DISORDERS THAT MAY RESULT*** *(see Specific Child Manifestation Clusters for additional information)* Oppositional defiant disorder (see p 119) Conduct disorder (p 119) Substance use/abuse (p 135) Generalized anxiety disorder (p 145) Posttraumatic stress disorder (p 145) Adjustment disorder (p 312) Depression (p 153) Somatoform disorder (p 173) Enuresis (p 215) Encopresis (p 219) Anorexia (p 227)/Bulimia (p 221) Insomnia (p 189)/Hypersomnia (p 181)

Table 3.

Environmental Situations and Potentially Stressful Events Checklist

Challenges to Primary Support Group V61.20
Challenges to Attachment Relationship **V61.20**
Death of a Parent or Other Family Member **V62.82**
Marital Discord **V61.1**
Divorce **V61.0**
Domestic Violence **V62.8**
Other Family Relationship Problems **V61.9**
Parent-Child Separation **V61.20**

Changes in Caregiving V61.20
Foster Care/Adoption/Institutional Care **V61.29**
Substance-Abusing Parents **V61.9**
Physical Abuse **995.54**
Sexual Abuse **995.53**
Quality of Nurture Problem **V61.20**
Neglect **995.52**
Mental Disorder of Parent **V61.8**
Physical Illness of Parent **V61.4**
Physical Illness of Sibling **V61.4**
Mental or Behavioral Disorder of Sibling **V61.8**

Other Functional Change in Family V61.2
Addition of a Sibling **V61.8**
Change in Parental Caregiver **V61.0**

Community or Social Challenges V62.4
Acculturation **V62.4**
Social Discrimination and/or Family Isolation **V62.81**
Religious or Spiritual Problem **V62.89**

Educational Challenges V62.3
Illiteracy of Parent **V62.3**
Inadequate School Facilities **V62.3**
Discord with Peers/Teachers **V62.3**

Parent or Adolescent Occupational Challenges V62.2
Unemployment **V62.0**
Loss of Job **V62.0**
Adverse Effect of Work Environment **V62.1**

Housing Challenges V60.0
Homelessness **V60.0**
Inadequate Housing **V60.1**
Unsafe Neighborhood **V60.8**
Dislocation **V60.8**

Economic Challenges V60.2
Poverty **V60.2**
Inadequate Financial Status **V60.2**

Inadequate Access to Health and/or Mental Health Services V61.9

Legal System or Crime Problem V62.5

Other Environmental Situations V62.8
Natural Disaster **V62.8**
Witness of Violence **V62.8**

Health-Related Situations V61.4
Chronic Health Conditions **V61.49**
Acute Health Conditions **V61.49**

Environmental Situations Defined

The codes, most of which are V codes, used in this listing were taken from the *ICD-9-CM*. Diagnoses should be listed in the order of importance, beginning with what first needs to be addressed. In some cases, one or more situations may be listed. General risk and protective factors of child and environment for all environmental situations are located in Table 1, p 36. Risk and protective factors are included under certain environmental events only when these vulnerabilities and strengths are known to be associated with these events.

Challenges to Primary Support Group

Changes in Caregiving

Other Functional Change in Family

Community or Social Challenges

Educational Challenges

Parent or Adolescent Occupational Challenges

Housing Challenges

Economic Challenges

Inadequate Access to Health and/or
    Mental Health Services

Legal System or Crime Problem

Other Environmental Situations

Health-Related Situations

Challenges to Attachment Relationship V61.20

Definition: Attachment refers to the affectionate and interactive ties that an infant forms with primary attachment figures (parent or caregiver). It is the emotional estrangement or physical separations that result in the loss of, or changes in, the availability and/or adequacy of the caregiver's capacity to support a child's development and emotional well-being. This may result from, for example, illness or hospitalization of attachment figures.

Risk Factors
- younger age (under the age of 4 years)
- poor coping by other primary attachment figures

Protective Factors
- older age (over the age of 4 years)
- presence of alternative, supportive attachment relationships

Death of a Parent or Other Family Member V62.82

Definition: An age-appropriate expression of significant emotional distress and a period of mourning following the death of a parent, primary caregiver, or other significant loved one are expected and should be anticipated. Child or adolescent behavioral symptoms following this major life event may reflect normal adaptation, symptomatic problems of adjustment, or the onset of a pathologic reaction to stress.

Risk Factors
- death of a parent before the child is 4 years of age
- mental disorders in the surviving parent
- preexisting behavioral problems
- poor adjustment of the family

Protective Factors
- older age with cognitive ability to comprehend the loss and mourning experience
- family system's increased capacity to balance need for emotional expression, mourning, and return to day-to-day routine, along with age-appropriate participation in effective "good-bye" rituals

Marital Discord V61.1/Divorce V61.0

Definition: Unresolved hostility, violence, or severe disagreement with or denigration of the partner. The children's parents alter their relationship so that the children's contact with either parent, or their perception of the stability and friendliness of the relationship may be substantially changed. This may involve separation after prolonged cohabitation or legal termination of the marriage.

Risk Factors

- close emotional relationship with the noncustodial parent
- childhood guilt about believing one is the cause of the marital discord
- sudden unexplained divorce
- greater hostility in divorce
- persistent conflict and litigation (particularly about custody)
- parental mental illness

Protective Factors

- consistent explanation and exoneration of the child
- absence of litigation/parental discord
- ongoing contact with both parents
- sparing children from the emotional conflict of the parents
- continued cooperation between parents to support the needs of the child

Domestic Violence V62.8

Definition: Situations in which parents or caregivers commit violent acts toward one another.

Risk Factors

- insecure attachment relationships
- caregiver's maladaptive reaction to stress
- difficult temperament
- inadequate family communication or marital conflict
- child perceives self as causing the abuse
- parental substance abuse
- chronic or recurrent health conditions

Protective Factors

- social competence
- positive family support and compensatory family caregivers
- high access to treatment resources

Other Family Relationship Problems V61.9

Many common situational problems present to primary care providers in the form of family relationship problems. Common presentations in this category include the following:

Parent-child problems such as problems in parent-child communication and conflicts. Parents may complain that the child does not adhere to rules and does not listen.

Sibling interaction problems such as persistent arguing and fighting, excessive competition, poor communication, and problems in adjusting to a sibling's special need or skills.

Parent-Child Separation V61.20

Definition: The physical separation of a child from parent, primary attachment relationship, or caregiver for any reason.

CHANGES IN CAREGIVING V61.20

Foster Care/Adoption/Institutional Care V61.29

Definition: The placement of a child by the legal system with primary providers other than their primary attachment relationship or caregiver, whether temporary, as in foster care, or permanent, as in adoption.

Substance Abusing Parents V61.8

Definition: The use of legal or illegal pharmacologic agents that affect the competence of primary care providers to provide adequate care to the children.

Physical Abuse 995.54/Sexual Abuse 995.53

Definition: Actions of adults that result in some form of direct physical or emotional harm to the child. Types include **physical** abuse or injury, **sexual** abuse in which the child is used for the purpose of sexual stimulation of an adult, and **emotional** or psychological abuse, defined as chronic hostility toward the child that is expressed in various forms such as rejecting, isolating, or terrorizing the child or in repeatedly holding the child responsible for negative events in the adult's life. *Factitious Disorder by Proxy* is a subtype of physical abuse in which a parent induces or fabricates a specific illness or physical or psychological symptom in an otherwise healthy child for the purpose of indirectly assuming the sick role.

Quality of Nurture Problem V61.20

Definition: Situations in which parents, primary care providers, or others, e.g., babysitters, do not provide adequate care. Examples of inadequate or problematic care of the child might include the following:
- inadequate supervision
- inadequate cognitive stimulation or emotional response
- repeated failure or inability to set appropriate limits on the child's behavior
- consistently harsh discipline or parenting practices
- highly inconsistent discipline or parenting practices
- parental overprotection
- "vulnerable child syndrome"

Neglect 995.52

Definition: The failure to provide basic physical care that adequately meets the child's needs for food and nutrition, failure to keep the child safe, failure to meet standards for preventive and/or acute medical care, and failure to meet community standards for emotional and cognitive nurturing. This inadequate caregiving differs from the other stressors in that it involves omissions or actions that compromise the child's physical and emotional well-being. Inadequate caregiving can occur in response to a specific event, such as parental job loss or marital discord, or it may reflect a chronic pattern of environmental insufficiency.

Risk Factors
- presence of other chronic stressors such as marital discord
- presence of physical or other abuse

Protective Factors
- compensatory family care providers
- unrelated positive adult role models

Mental Disorder of Parent V61.8

Definition: Situations in which parents or primary caregivers have mental disorders or problems that negatively affect their ability to provide adequate nurture, care, and stimulation for their children.

Physical Illness of Parent V61.4

Definition: Situations in which parents or primary caregivers have acute or chronic health conditions that affect their ability to provide care, nurture, or stimulation for their children.

Physical Illness of Sibling V61.4

Definition: Situations in which siblings experience acute or chronic health problems that place significant burdens on family members.

Mental or Behavioral Disorder of Sibling V61.8

Definition: Situations in which siblings experience behavioral or mental disorders that place significant burdens on family members.

OTHER FUNCTIONAL CHANGE IN FAMILY V61.2

Addition of a Sibling V61.8

Definition: The addition of a sibling to the family by birth, adoption, or blending. This change can have beneficial effects such as enhancing social, play, and coping skills and increasing the self-esteem of children who both give and receive nurturing. The addition of a sibling can also be stressful.

Risk Factors
- absence of compensatory caregivers
- family discord
- physical/emotional exhaustion in parents
- housing circumstances problem

Protective Factors
- a prior secure pattern of attachment
- good marital relationship
- adequate support available from the parent and other compensatory care providers

Change in Parental Caregiver V61.0

Definition: Many families experience significant changes in parental caregivers, e.g., the addition of stepparents through remarriage. In other instances, parents or other family caregivers may now be absent from the home owing to changes in their employment status, divorce, military service, or incarceration.

COMMUNITY OR SOCIAL CHALLENGES V62.4

Acculturation V62.4

Definition: A situation involving adjustment to a different culture, most commonly involving immigration.

Social Discrimination and/or Family Isolation V62.81

Religious or Spiritual Problem V62.89

Definition: Situations in which problems regarding religious or spiritual matters exist, including stressful experiences that involve loss or questioning of faith, problems associated with conversion to a new faith, or questioning of spiritual values that may not necessarily be related to any organized church or religious institution.

EDUCATIONAL CHALLENGES V62.3

Definition: Educational issues that are not due to mental problems or disorders.

Illiteracy of Parent V62.3

Definition: A situation in which parents are unable to read.

Inadequate School Facilities V62.3

Definition: A situation in which children are not provided with adequate school facilities.

Discord With Peers/Teachers V62.3

Definition: A situation in which there are major disagreements with peers/teachers.

Parent or Adolescent Occupational Challenges V62.2

Parent Occupational Challenges V62.2

Definition: A situation in which a parent is experiencing an occupational problem that is creating stress for the child.

Adolescent Occupational Challenges V62.2

Definition: A situation in which an adolescent is experiencing an occupational problem (e.g., in a current job or with regard to career choice) that is not due to a mental disorder, or, if due to a mental disorder, warrants independent clinical attention.

Unemployment V62.0

Definition: A situation in which a parents are unemployed.

Loss of Job V62.0

Definition: A situation in which parents have lost employment.

Adverse Effect of Work Environment V62.1

Definition: A situation in which an adolescent or parent is experiencing an adverse work environment.

HOUSING CHALLENGES V60.0

Homelessness V60.0

Definition: In the pediatric population, homelessness includes children who live with families who have no permanent living situation and runaway adolescents. Families with children, the fastest growing segment of the homeless population, represent a large percentage of the homeless population and nearly half of the homeless population in large urban settings.

Risk Factors
◆ exposure to violence
◆ substance abuse
◆ poor access to services

Protective Factors
◆ nurturing and supportive parent/child attachment relationships

Inadequate Housing V60.1

Definition: Refers to housing that is substandard and exposes the child to risks, e.g., lead poisoning.

Unsafe Neighborhood V60.8

Definition: A situation in which a child's neighborhood has a high rate of crime and violence.

Dislocation V60.8

Definition: A condition in which the family loses its home and is forced to move into other living circumstances. Occasionally symptoms will result even when the household move is planned.

ECONOMIC CHALLENGES V60.2

Poverty/Inadequate Financial Status V60.2

Definition: Federal guidelines define poverty at specific income levels that vary according to the year and the number of people in the household. Living in poverty is a chronic contextual situation that increases the likelihood of behavioral symptoms and disorders. Poverty is not usually a direct etiologic agent. Although most children who live in poverty develop normally, possible mechanisms that increase the likelihood of mental problems and disorders exist, including a greater chance of biological and nutritional problems in the child, and a greater chance of having a deficiency in caregiving environment, including more stress, less stability and organization, and less access to services. In 1992, 21.8% of all children between the ages of 6 to 17 years old and 26% of all children younger than 6 years lived in poverty.

INADEQUATE ACCESS TO HEALTH AND/OR MENTAL HEALTH SERVICES V61.9

Definition: A situation in which children live in circumstances where health and mental health services are physically not available, or the family is not able to access these services because of transportation problems or problems in paying for such services.

LEGAL SYSTEM OR CRIME PROBLEM V62.5

Crime Problem of Parent

Definition: A situation in which a child's parent is significantly involved with the legal system due to arrest, incarceration, or victimization by crime.

Juvenile Crime Problem V62.5

Definition: A situation in which a child or adolescent is significantly involved with the legal system due to arrest, incarceration, or probation.

OTHER ENVIRONMENTAL SITUATIONS V62.8

Natural Disaster V62.8

Definition: Situations such as hurricanes, floods, or tornadoes caused by nature that disrupt normal activities.

Witness of Violence V62.8

Definition: Situations in which individuals witness or are victims of street or community violence. Visualizing simulated violence, as in movies and on television, may have a negative impact, but the effect is generally not as severe as being a victim or a witness of actual violence.

HEALTH-RELATED SITUATIONS V61.4

Chronic Health Conditions V61.49

Definition: Chronic health conditions include physical illnesses or impairments that have lasted, or are expected to last, more than 3 months. Many conditions, especially more severe ones, limit age-appropriate school, play, and recreational activities, and require medical attention greater than that expected for a child of the same age. Physical illnesses and impairments have an impact on the psychological functioning of children and create predictable demands and burdens for families. These effects are not limited to the actual disease or impairment, but also include the diagnostic procedures and treatments that may set the occasion for particular responses.

Estimates of the number of children with chronic physical disorders vary from 10% to 30% of the total population, with physiologically severe conditions affecting 2% to 4% of all children. Some chronic illnesses represent adaptational challenges that may require the psychological intervention of primary care providers on a recurring basis.

Risk Factors

- negative responses of family: isolation, anger, and inappropriate protectiveness, restrictions, or expectations
- family dysfunction
- difficult child temperament

Protective Factors

- supportive family responses (e.g., love, friendship)
- provision of information, advice, and physical comfort
- intervention provided by primary care providers
- relatively brief, specific interventions, such as educational programs, counseling, or behavior management

Acute Health Conditions V61.49

Definition: Acute health conditions involve a transient health episode or impairment that serves as a stressor for the child's or parent's functioning or mental health. Examples include self-limited viral illness, a nonserious fracture, or a burn. Some acute but recurrent health conditions, such as recurrent otitis media or sinusitis, may produce recurrent stress comparable to a chronic health condition and should be so classified. Some conditions may develop into chronic health conditions, such as varicella followed by encephalitis. An atypical response to an acute health condition is a useful clue to underlying, perhaps unrecognized, child, family, or community problems. Consider Factitious Disorder by Proxy. It is not unusual for infants and young children to have many acute health episodes in one calendar year, especially in large families or out-of-home care.

Risk Factors

- difficult child temperament
- family dysfunction
- unsupportive community

Protective Factors

- easy (good fit) child temperament
- positive family function
- supportive community
- flexible child care opportunities

CHILD MANIFESTATIONS
SECTION

This classification was developed with the recognition that behaviors throughout development are a reflection of complex interactions between environmental influences and characteristics of the child's developing neurological system. However, this section of the nomenclature emphasizes the individual behaviors and the behavioral clusters (i.e., syndromes) that are demonstrated by the child. These behaviors can be thought of as "intrinsic" to the child, although clear distinctions between behaviors intrinsic to the child and those representing a reaction to events outside the child are difficult to make.

Support for the biological basis of these behaviors is sometimes clear. Certain behaviors, for example, occur in the majority of children in association with a particular phase of development across cultures. Examples include the wariness of strangers that appears in most infants between 7 and 10 months of age, or the negativism typical of toddlers at around the age of 2 years. The neurological basis for other behaviors is inferred from their association with known neuropathology such as the cognitive-perceptual deficits associated with temporal lobe lesions in the brain or the dysarthria associated with cerebral palsy.

Often, however, the intrinsic nature of behaviors or behavioral syndromes is based on less clear evidence. Such evidence would include the appearance of the behavior early in the child's life when environmental factors have had less of a chance to have an effect, or behaviors where familial patterns are present.

Clearly, however, all these so-called intrinsic behaviors are influenced by events in the child's life, interactions with important others, and specific stressors such as child abuse or the death of a close family member.

The behaviors in this section are organized into categories of child manifestations that are based on the similarities of the behaviors or the disorders that result when those behaviors are severe. The categories include:

1. Developmental competencies such as learning ability, motor skills, and academic skills, and speech and language

2. Impulsive, hyperactive, and inattentive behaviors that are grouped together because of their impact on school performance and their appearance as a common syndrome indicating a disorder (i.e., attention-deficit/hyperactivity disorder)

3. Negative and antisocial behaviors that are grouped together because of their similar impact on caregivers and others in the child's life

4. Substance use and/or abuse, which includes a complex set of behaviors not easily categorized elsewhere

5. Emotions and moods, behaviors that are usually seen as emotional in nature

6. Somatic behavior, including sleep, that is usually associated with bodily symptoms

7. Feeding, eating, and elimination behaviors that are related by their common origin in ingestion

8. Illness-related behaviors that are grouped together because they all involve responses to illness (e.g., compliance issues)

9. Sexual behaviors that are related to sexuality at different stages of development

10. Atypical behaviors that are seen as unusual or bizarre

Each of these categories includes one or more **clusters** of presenting complaints — the statements typically made by caregivers or other adults when they express concern about that behavior. Each behavioral cluster is described and instructions are given for identifying the behaviors as normal developmental variants, problems, or disorders. Even when the child's behavior represents normal variation, it may be a cause of concern. Reasons for those concerns may be quite varied, ranging from parents who are stressed by problems of their own to environmental concerns such as poverty that may make the behaviors a problem for that family. At this time, the code provided by the developmental variation categories of the manual is V65.49, a nonspecific *ICD-9-CM* counseling code. When the behaviors occur at a level considered to be a problem or a disorder, they are likely to have a negative impact both on the child and important others in the child's environment. It is important that these behaviors are categorized and receive intervention. Currently the problems have been assigned an *ICD-9-CM* problem code.

When the behavior is severe enough to be considered a disorder, the label and diagnostic criteria for that disorder, already categorized in the *Diagnostic and Statistical Manual of Mental Disorders (DSM-IV)*, are used.

Children may have more than one child manifestation unless the instructions specify that one diagnosis takes precedent. This has been referred to as comorbidity.

DEVELOPMENTAL COMPETENCY

COGNITIVE/ADAPTIVE SKILLS
(MENTAL RETARDATION) CLUSTER

ACADEMIC SKILLS CLUSTER

MOTOR DEVELOPMENT CLUSTER

SPEECH AND LANGUAGE CLUSTER

Cognitive/Adaptive Skills (Mental Retardation)

Presenting Complaints

unusual appearance (head too large or small or deformed)

not yet walking

not yet talking

still talking baby talk

does not avoid hazards

not feeding or dressing self yet

not yet toilet trained

does not remember things

failing in school

unable to keep a job or do what is expected at home

Definitions and Symptoms

Mental retardation is defined by a child's significant below-average progress in the development of his or her cognitive abilities and adaptive behaviors. Although the assessment of general intellectual abilities is frequently categorized by a single intellectual quotient, it is misleading to conceptualize intelligence as a single trait. Intelligence as it is measured includes a number of different areas such as memory, vocabulary, conceptual thinking, computational skills, perceptions of patterns, and the association of concepts. More recent emphasis has been placed on adaptive skills as important aspects. The relationship between mental retardation and learning disorders entails differences both in severity and in the pattern of skill strengths and deficits. For many children with mental retardation the deficits are more global but varying patterns are also observed.

In early infancy, it is not yet possible to predict cognitive development behaviorally. Thus, a firm prediction of mental retardation in a fetus or young infant is not feasible though the presence of some medical conditions is clearly associated with high risk (e.g., the presence of a chromosomal anomaly, an inborn error of metabolism, or a specific dysmorphic syndrome likely to be associated with mental retardation). The more severe forms of mental retardation are evident as a delay in early developmental milestones such as walking, talking, feeding and dressing self, and toilet training, yet most children with delayed milestones in any one area develop normally or have more specific difficulties such as motor or language problems. The milder forms of mental retardation may not become evident until the child experiences difficulty in preschool or school. Again, however, most children with early academic difficulties may have variations in learning style or learning disorders rather than mental retardation. On the other hand, some children with mental retardation have other major disorders such as autism or pervasive developmental disorder (see Social Interaction Behaviors cluster, p 277).

Epidemiology

The prevalence rate of mental retardation has been estimated at approximately 2% to 3%. The majority (85% to 90%) fall at the mild level. However, different studies have reported different rates depending on definitions used, methods of ascertainment, and population studied. Mental retardation is more common in males with a male-to-female ratio of approximately 1.5:1.

Etiology

Literally hundreds of possible etiological causes of mental retardation have been identified. Nevertheless, recent epidemiological research suggests that in about 30% of children with severe mental retardation, the etiology is unknown. The same is true in about 50% of the children with mild mental retardation. It is often not possible to attribute a particular child's retardation to a single cause; in up to half of the children in which causal factors are known, there is more than one such factor, for example, low birth weight and lack of intellectual stimulation in the home. Malnutrition and certain toxins such as alcohol or lead can adversely affect brain development before or after birth and thus cause mental retardation.

DEVELOPMENTAL VARIATION	COMMON DEVELOPMENTAL PRESENTATIONS

V65.4 Developmental/ Cognitive Variation

There is a wide range of variation in the ages at which different milestones are reached, whether in the areas of language and communication, motor skills, self-help skills, or academic and vocational accomplishments. Clinicians can use parental concerns and/or formal screening procedures to make judgments that a child's cognitive development is within these broad limits.

Infancy

The child walks or talks toward the end of the expected age range. Motor and language skills may show considerable variation. There is relatively less expectable variation in the infant's general ability to show increasing relatedness and increasing intentionality (via gestures such as looking, pointing, vocalizing, reciprocal vocalizing, frowning, etc.) in the 6- to 12-month range when it should be increasing.

Early Childhood

The child acquires skills at the upper end of age expectations. A common landmark with a wide variation is toilet training.

Middle Childhood and Adolescence

Problems arise in children of average capabilities if they are placed in environments with unrealistic expectations.

SPECIAL INFORMATION

Generally, infants do not begin to walk or talk until about 12 months of age, and many are late in developing these skills without any dire prognostic implications. During the course of early childhood, children usually learn to speak intelligibly in sentences, learn to feed and dress themselves, and are successfully toilet trained. Once more, there are wide normal variations in the times at which these milestones are accomplished. Children who attend school in the United States can be expected to begin to learn to read by the end of the 1st grade. By the end of elementary school, they should have acquired the basics of reading, writing, spelling, and simple arithmetic well enough to use these skills in more advanced academic work. Teenagers are expected to progress through middle school and high school and to become capable of paid employment.

Developmental inventories provide a convenient list of developmental milestones together with normative information so that a preliminary estimate can be made of whether a particular child's development is delayed. However, the early items on such inventories have a heavy sensory-motor component and cannot in themselves be regarded as cognitive skills. The child can be followed over time, which can enhance the accuracy over one observation or assessment. Parental concern about developmental delays should be considered seriously. They may overdiagnose conditions but their accuracy in many cases is better than clinical judgment without formal screening. More extensive assessment may be available through the public school or through state early intervention programs.

PROBLEM	COMMON DEVELOPMENTAL PRESENTATIONS
V62.3 Developmental/ Cognitive Problem In the cognitive/adaptive domain, a "problem" exists when the child is significantly behind in achieving any milestones according to the clinician's subjective norms or formal screening criteria, to the extent that the delay causes some practical difficulty in the child's life. This is categorized as Borderline intellectual functioning (**V62.89**) in older children.	**Infancy** The child may show mild delays such as walking or talking beyond expected normal range, but in many cases may have normal development. Recent evidence suggests that the lack of two-way communication (reciprocation of gestures such as smile, frown, sound, motor patterning — pointing or taking object from caregiver) or the baby's inability to indicate wants are strongly suggestive of some cognitive delays. **Early Childhood** The child may show similar characteristics to those described for academic skills problem. The child experiences delays in recognition of alphabetic and numeric symbols, shapes, colors, sounds, symbol associations, has poor preliteracy skills. **Middle Childhood and Adolescence** The child is unable to make adequate progress in academic tasks and social adaptations.

SPECIAL INFORMATION
A formal assessment is usually necessary to conclude that an infant is significantly behind in developmental milestones. For children under 5, assessment is available in most states through the early intervention programs. Early identification is important to identify affected children as early as possible to enroll them in early intervention programs. The cognitive development of a child who "fails" academically or has to repeat a grade should be evaluated. Consistently poor grades in school are reason to evaluate cognitive/ adaptive development.

DISORDER	COMMON DEVELOPMENTAL PRESENTATIONS
317, 318.x, 319 Mental Retardation Significantly subaverage intellectual functioning is found: an IQ score of approximately 70 or below on an individually administered IQ test (for infants, a clinical judgment of significantly subaverage intellectual functioning). Mental retardation is coded based on degree of severity: **317.** Mild mental retardation (IQ level 50-55 to approximately 70) **318.0** Moderate mental retardation (IQ level 35-40 to 50-55) **318.1** Severe mental retardation (IQ level 20-25 to 35-40) **318.2** Profound mental retardation (IQ level below 20 to 25) **319.** Mental retardation severity unspecified is diagnosed when there is a strong presumption of mental retardation but the child's intelligence is untestable by standard intelligence tests. In addition, the child or adolescent shows concurrent deficits or limitations in present adaptive skills functioning (the person's effectiveness in meeting the standards expected for his or her age by his or her cultural group) in at least two of the following adaptive skill areas: communication, self-care, home living, social skills, community youth resources, self-direction, functional academic skills, work, leisure, health, and safety. The onset is before the age of 18 years.	**Infancy** The infant, particularly with moderate or severe deficits, has significant limitations in emotional expressiveness, language, purposeful behavior, gross/fine motor skills (see Motor Development cluster, p 77), and assessed cognitive limitations including language delays. Mild deficits may go undetected. **Early Childhood** The child has significant limitations in communication, walking, self-feeding, toileting, and social interaction, and has significant subaverage intellectual function. **Middle Childhood and Adolescence** The delays in development by this age are usually clear and evaluation can identify strengths and weaknesses in cognitive and adaptive abilities. **SPECIAL INFORMATION** In implementing the definition of mental retardation (as summarized in the adjacent column under "Disorder," the American Association of Mental Retardation in the 1992 Definition, Classification, and System of Supports suggests that the following four assumptions are essential to the application of the definition: Valid assessment considers cultural and linguistic diversity as well as differences in communication and behavioral factors. The existence of limitations in adaptive skills occurs within the context of community environments typical of the individual's age peers and is indexed to the person's individualized needs for supports. Specific adaptive limitations often coexist with strengths in other adaptive skills or other personal capabilities. With appropriate supports over a sustained period, the life functioning of the person with mental retardation will generally improve.

	SPECIAL INFORMATION, CONTINUED
	The above-referenced 1992 system also suggests the following three-step process that focuses on diagnosis for intervention planning.
	Step 1: The diagnosis of mental retardation (see adjacent column).
	Step 2: The identification of strengths and limitations across the four dimensions of: (1) intellectual functioning and adaptive skills, (2) psychological and emotional considerations, (3) physical health/etiology considerations, and (4) environmental considerations.
	Step 3: The profiling of the types and intensities of needed supports across the four dimensions given in step 2.
	Intensity of needed supports are defined as:
	Intermittent: Supports on an "as needed basis." Characterized by episodic nature, person not always needing the support(s), or short-term supports needed during life-span transitions.
	————
	The criteria for mental retardation are in a state of flux. The criteria as stated in the top paragraph and listed in the left-hand column reflect the *DSM-IV* criteria with undefined deficits in adaptive behavior. The American Association of Mental Retardation is now recommending a requirement of IQ testing of 70 to 75 and the addition of the adaptive deficits as outlined in the bottom paragraph in the left-hand column. The new criteria are currently being debated and consensus has not yet been established. Assessments have to be sensitive to cultural diversity and other deficits such as sensory or motor impairments.

DIFFERENTIAL DIAGNOSIS	SPECIAL INFORMATION
General Medical Conditions — Examples include: Phenylketonuria Fragile X syndrome Down's syndrome	The list of medical syndromes involving mental retardation is too extensive to be given here in detail. A diagnosis of mental retardation should be made even if a medical condition is present.
Substances — Examples include: Alcohol Lead	Certain toxins such as alcohol (prenatal) or lead (prenatal or postnatal) can adversely affect brain development before or after birth and thus cause mental retardation.
Mental Disorders **299.00** Autistic disorder **315.00** Reading disorder **315.1** Mathematics disorder **315.2** Disorder of written expression **315.31** Expressive language disorder **315.39** Phonological disorder	Many children with autistic disorder or another pervasive developmental disorder function in the range of mental retardation. IQ range for borderline intellectual functioning is generally 71 to 84; however, an IQ score may involve a measurement error of approximately 5 points, depending on the testing instrument.

COMMONLY COMORBID CONDITIONS	SPECIAL INFORMATION
Other Comorbid Mental Health Conditions — Examples include: 314.01 Attention-deficit/hyperactivity disorder combined type 314.01 Attention-deficit/hyperactivity disorder predominantly hyperactive-impulsive type 314.00 Attention-deficit/hyperactivity disorder predominantly inattentive type 300.02 Generalized anxiety disorder 296.xx Major depressive disorder 300.3 Obsessive-compulsive disorder 299.00 Autistic disorder 307.3 Stereotypic movement disorder Mental disorders due to a general medical condition	Individuals with mental retardation may be vulnerable to exploitation by others (being physically and sexually abused). It is estimated that individuals with mental retardation have a prevalence of comorbid mental disorders that is estimated to be four times greater than the prevalence in the general population.
Other General Medical Conditions — Examples include: Cerebral palsy Hydrocephalus/spina bifida Epilepsy Down's syndrome	Approximately half of those with cerebral palsy have significant mental retardation. Children with hydrocephalus/spina bifida and epilepsy are at higher risk for retardation as a result of their neurological conditions but the clinician should not assume impairment based on the general medical condition. In severe or profound mental retardation, there is a greater likelihood of neurological (seizures), neuromuscular, visual, auditory, or cardiovascular conditions. If mental retardation is associated with other conditions, consider coding injury-induced mental retardation, or mental retardation secondary to a neurosensory condition.

Presenting Complaints

poor test scores/poor grades
"underachieving"
not learning or retaining skills well
slower than other kids
repeating a grade

Definitions and Symptoms

The childhood years are characterized by the steady acquisition of knowledge. From the first glimmers of distinguishing the human face to the "ah hah" at understanding differential calculus, children learn to read signals and symbols, to count and compute, and to express themselves in written and spoken language. Along the childhood pathway, all children experience some areas of learning that are more difficult than others and most excel in one or another sphere. For some children there are areas that become truly problematic, setting them back, and causing distress and concern. These problems can generally be overcome by targeted intervention, allowing the child to progress with little or no further input. If, however, the child is actually deficient in the basic processes that facilitate reading, writing, and computing, and if intervention is always needed to assure progress, the child is said to have a specific disorder in reading, writing, or mathematics. Difficulties in learning manifest themselves in a wide variety of ways. Children with academic skills problems may first come to the attention of their schools and parents because they cannot manage the day-to-day school tasks, or some children may struggle by — just reaching an acceptable threshold of performance. In either of these cases, the first sign of trouble may come as a related behavior problem (forgetting to do homework assignments, acting out, refusing to go to school, withdrawing, displaying inattention or a lack of persistence), in which the learning problem is primary and the behavioral difficulties are secondary. On the other hand, children with emotional and/or behavioral problems (e.g., from emotional disorders [see Sadness and Related symptoms, p 153], attention-deficit/hyperactivity disorder [see Hyperactive/Impulsive Behaviors cluster, p 93], posttraumatic stress disorder [see Anxious Symptoms cluster, p 145]) can present with poor school performance as a major manifestation of their situation. It is essential that the primary care physician be alert to the broad array of comorbidities associated with learning problems.

Epidemiology

Estimates of the prevalence of learning disorders range from 2% to 10% depending on the nature of ascertainment and the definition applied. Approximately 5% of the students in public schools in the United States are identified as having a learning disorder, although this may reflect the criteria that have been preset by the schools.

Etiology

Academic skills deficits may be inherited or secondary to CNS insults (e.g., prematurity with pulmonary involvement, closed head injury, lead poisoning, fetal alcohol syndrome, and fragile X syndrome).

DEVELOPMENTAL VARIATION	COMMON DEVELOPMENTAL PRESENTATIONS

V65.49 Learning Variation

Learning styles vary enormously among children and are reflected in differences in the rate, quality, retention, analysis, and application of what is learned. Some children learn quickly. Others require extensive repetition of material before it is retained. Some children learn best through the auditory route; others learn best visually. Similarly, children vary as to the strength of their verbal vs written responses. The method of instruction may enhance or detract from the child's ability to learn the material(s) presented.

Infancy
Developmental delays in this age group are essentially the same as described in the developmental/cognitive variation (infancy section, p 63).

Early Childhood
The child likes puzzles, block building, sorting, categorizing, understands concepts of big/little, up/down, back/front, understands less/more, processes one- and two-step instructions, follows "rules" in group games and activities, listens to stories, follows along in picture books, questions "what," "where," "when," and "how." Parents begin to worry about learning problems if their child does not progress at the same rate as age-equivalent peers.

Middle Childhood
The child understands left/right and follows print from left-to-right on a page, learns symbolic representations (letters, numbers), writes, advances in quantitative ability (adding, subtracting, multiplying, dividing), understands and uses jokes/humor.

Adolescence
Adolescents develop special interests, begin future planning, demonstrate variability in skill levels, and develop a fuller understanding of abstract material in later years.

SPECIAL INFORMATION

In infancy, learning is largely a reciprocal activity with parents (and other adults) and may vary in richness depending on the exposure of the child to a developmentally appropriate and language-rich environment. Measures of home environment can assist the clinician in documenting the degree to which this environment promotes developmental attainment and early learning.

In early childhood, variability occurs in the rate of acquisition of school readiness skills (e.g., learning songs and nursery rhymes and other rote activities such as reciting the alphabet and counting numbers); in the range of abilities to use materials such as crayons, chalk, and pencils; and in the range of family stimulation from occasional to nightly bedtime reading. The extent to which parents and day care providers read to children and introduce them to preliterate experiences are strong predictors of children's academic success.

In middle childhood, some parents and teachers have unrealistic expectations of the child's abilities. This is particularly true of high-achieving parents. A child's comfort with subject areas and teaching methods varies. Some children are particularly gifted in one or more academic areas. Assessments of a child's rate of learning and academic expectations should be based on objective information. The clinician should review the results of IQ and achievement tests and review the child's report cards before clarifying expectations.

In adolescence, academic achievement varies with interest and skill preferences. Early choices may be made regarding vocation. Competing interests such as work for pay, sports, clubs, and extracurricular activities may impinge on the academic interest and performance of teenagers. Also, performance may be impaired by developmental norms such as experimentation with alcohol or other drugs (see Substance Use/Abuse cluster, p 135), preoccupation with sexual relationships (see Sexual Development Behaviors cluster, p 261), and lack of appreciation for future consequences.

PROBLEM	COMMON DEVELOPMENTAL PRESENTATIONS
V40.0 Learning Problem All children have neurodevelopmental strengths and weaknesses. For some children, the areas of weakness begin to affect their ability to learn and function in the academic environment. These difficulties are often transient, particularly if they are promptly recognized and afforded appropriate targeted interventions.	**Infancy** The presentation of learning problems do not appear as a separate entity from cognitive developmental problems in this age group. **Early Childhood** The child experiences delays in recognition of alphabetic and numeric symbols, shapes, colors, sounds, symbol associations, and has poor preliteracy skills. In early childhood, a child should recognize and reproduce shapes (cross, circle, square) by age 4 years. A child should be able to recite the alphabet and recognize colors by age 4½ to 5 years and write at least ABCD and rote count to 20 by age 5 years. Delays are limited to those actions that are precursors of academic activities. **Middle Childhood** The child generally underachieves, has inconsistent academic performance from term to term, occasionally does poorly in some subjects, evinces mild to moderate lack of interest in school. **Adolescence** The adolescent has weak reading skills, has problems with homework, has organizational difficulties, fails certain subject areas, has poor written and verbal skills but does not qualify for having an academic disorder.

SPECIAL INFORMATION

In infancy, the sensorimotor period described by Piaget extends from birth to 18 months. Conceptual frames of reference are established by young children during this period. In the 0- to 2-month period, critical cognitive and conceptual skills begin to emerge. If the child is thwarted in attempting to explore and make sense of the world, this can be a problem. Understimulating environments (see quality of nurture problem, p 46) present a hazard in this regard. Also, children who have sensory and/or motor problems may not experience the outside world as clearly as their peers do.

Delays in learning may occur because parents do not read to the child.

In middle childhood, obtain the child's IQ and achievement data. Look for changes in the child's school environment — smaller to larger class size, a different type of teacher, move from homeroom to changing classes, or a heavier homework load. A new school, new neighborhood, or new sports or extracurricular commitment may also affect learning.

In adolescence, consider social pressures and expectations. Take a careful social, sexual, and substance use history. How are academics viewed in the teen culture? Are good grades looked down upon by peers?

Family stresses such as marital discord (see p 44), moves, or poverty/inadequate financial status (see p 51) can exacerbate learning problems by causing a child to be preoccupied with these events and less receptive to learning new facts and skills.

Lack of resources (books, libraries) can have a major influence on school readiness and school performance.

Child/teacher mismatch can account for some transient school performance problems. They can also be related to stressful events or issues, such as chronic health condition (see p 52), which can also contribute to the problem through frequent school absences.

DISORDER	COMMON DEVELOPMENTAL PRESENTATIONS

315.00 Reading Disorder (developmental reading disorder)

Reading achievement, as measured by individually administered standardized tests of reading accuracy or comprehension, substantially below that expected given the person's chronological age, measured intelligence, and age-appropriate education. The reading disturbance significantly interferes with academic achievement or activities of daily living that require reading skills. If a sensory deficit is present, the reading difficulties are in excess of those usually associated with it.

315.1 Mathematics Disorder (developmental arithmetic disorder)

Mathematical ability, as measured by individually administered standardized tests, is substantially below that expected given the person's chronological age, measured intelligence, and age-appropriate education. The disturbance significantly interferes with academic achievement or activities of daily living that require mathematical ability. If a sensory deficit is present, the difficulties in mathematical ability are in excess of those associated with it.

315.2 Disorder of Written Expression (developmental expressive writing disorder)

Writing skills, as measured by individually administered standardized tests (or functional assessment of writing skills), are substantially below that expected given the person's chronological age, measured intelligence, and age-appropriate education. The disturbance significantly interferes with academic achievement or activities of daily living that require the composition of written texts (e.g., writing grammatically correct sentences and organized paragraphs). If a sensory deficit is present, the difficulties in writing skills are in excess of those usually associated with it.

Infancy
Not relevant at this age.

Early Childhood
The child is unable to do simple puzzles, does not sort, count, categorize, shows no understanding of simple concepts (big/little), does not follow instructions, cannot remember routines. However, it is difficult to make a definitive diagnosis in this age group.

Middle Childhood
The child with a reading disorder cannot read words by 7 years of age, does not associate sounds with letters, has difficulty with word attack, decoding, blending, or fluency of reading, and word identification, has difficulty with reading comprehension and poor spelling, has problems in composition including narration, organization, grammar, punctuation, capitalization. The child with a mathematics disorder does not acquire computational skills (adding, subtracting, etc.) and may show difficulty with making change or understanding concepts such as time. The child with a written expression disorder will have difficulties in constructing sentences and paragraphs.

Adolescence
The adolescent can have a serious reading disability and an inability to express thoughts in writing, inability to use quantitative skills in a functional manner, or a combination of these deficits. These can result in their not understanding subjects such as social studies and history or having difficulties with foreign language acquisition.

SPECIAL INFORMATION

It is not possible to decide that an infant has an academic skills disorder. Infants who are suspected of having serious developmental delays should be monitored through early intervention programs. Infants and young children with disorders in language (see Speech and Language cluster, p 83), cognitive abilities (see Cognitive/ Adaptive Skills cluster, p 61), and/or motor skills (see Motor Development cluster, p 77) are at high risk for later academic skills problems and/or disorders.

In early childhood, educational programs such as Head Start are appropriate for children who evince signs of preacademic difficulty. It is important to clarify a child's hearing and vision status when there are concerns with learning.

Younger children may present with a constellation of findings that have been correlated with later reading, writing, and math problems. These include poor naming skills, difficulty learning colors and quantitative concepts (greater/lesser, bigger/smaller, one-to-one correspondence and counting). These children should be considered to have preacademic problems that warrant careful monitoring and specific intervention when appropriate.

The diagnosis usually requires assessment of the child by qualified professionals in psychology and education. In many cases this is provided by school systems but external second opinions are sometimes helpful.

In middle childhood, when children have serious and sustained academic difficulty, obtain IQ, achievement data, a report card, and parent/teacher ratings for the evaluation of possible inattention. Check

	SPECIAL INFORMATION, CONTINUED
315.9 Learning Disorder, NOS	the child's visual acuity and hearing. Truancy in the middle childhood years is a strong correlate with lifetime learning problems. Truants should be evaluated carefully for signs of learning disorders. In adolescence, the same disorders should be considered as in middle childhood. If the onset of problems occurs in adolescence, consider the potential contribution of factors such as substance abuse (see Substance Use/Abuse cluster, p 135), anxiety and post-traumatic stress disorder (see Anxious Symptoms cluster, p 145), mood disorders (see Sadness Symptoms clusters, p 153), and/or other psychosocial stressors such as problems of primary support group (see p 43) and educational circumstances (see p 48). It is often difficult to distinguish learning disorders from other mental disorders or problems.

DIFFERENTIAL DIAGNOSIS	SPECIAL INFORMATION
General Medical Conditions— Examples include: Chronic illnesses that have direct effects on the CNS such as human immuno-deficiency virus infection Traumatic injury Prematurity Neurobiologic conditions (neurofibromatosis) Chromosomal abnormalities (Turner, Klinefelter, Fragile X syndromes) CNS syndromes such as Riley-Day syndrome Postinfections Postchemotherapy Lead poisoning/other heavy metals	Missed school days may set a child back in specific areas. Impaired vision or hearing may affect learning ability and should be investigated through audiometric or visual screening tests. If a sensory deficit is present, a learning disorder can still be diagnosed, but only if the learning difficulties are in excess of the learning difficulties that would usually be associated with that sensory deficit. An acute decrease in a child's school functioning should increase one's suspicion of a general medical condition or a mental disorder.
Substances — Examples include: Alcohol Marijuana Cocaine Prenatal drug/alcohol exposure Medications: Anticholinergics Benzodiazepine	Dramatic, acute changes in school performance should cause concern and raise the possibility of drug/alcohol use.
Mental Disorders **315.xx,** Communication disorders **307.xx** **317,** Mental retardation **318.x,** **319** **299.00** Autistic disorder **V62.89** Borderline intellectual functioning **314.xx** Attention-deficit/hyperactivity disorder **296.xx** Major depressive disorder **300.02** Generalized anxiety disorder	Mental retardation is usually, but not always, diagnosed before age 7 years (see Cognitive/Adaptive Skills cluster, p 61). Mental retardation can present as an academic skills disorder. However, general abilities are in the range of mental retardation, there are deficits in adaptive skills, and a significant discrepancy does not exist between general abilities and academic performance. Developmental/cognitive problems (borderline intellectual ability, p 64) may present as a skills disorder. Learning disorders must be differentiated from normal variations in academic attainment and from scholastic difficulties due to lack of opportunity, poor teaching, and cultural factors.

COMMONLY COMORBID CONDITIONS	SPECIAL INFORMATION
Other Comorbid Mental Health Conditions — Examples include: **309.21** Separation anxiety disorder/school phobia **314.xx** Attention-deficit/hyperactivity disorder **296.xx** Major depressive disorder **300.4** Dysthymic disorder **313.81** Oppositional defiant disorder **312.81** Conduct disorder childhood onset **312.82** Conduct disorder adolescent onset **315.4** Developmental coordination disorder **315.xx, 307.xx** Communication disorders **317, 318.x, 319** Mental retardation	These conditions can be causes of academic difficulties or they can be comorbid conditions. If treatment of these disorders results in significant amelioration of the academic problem or disorder, the relationship is likely to be causal. Mental retardation and academic disorder can occur together if there is still a significant discrepancy between general abilities and academic performance.
Other General Medical Conditions — Examples include: Lead poisoning Fetal alcohol syndrome Fragile X syndrome CNS insults (e.g., prematurity with pulmonary involvement, closed head injury)	Not relevant.

Presenting Complaints

motor delay ("not walking")

clumsiness

incoordination

poor handwriting

poor athletic performance

Definition and Symptoms

Gross motor development is typically monitored closely by parents and primary care physicians during the early years of life primarily because of the relative ease with which gross motor milestones can be observed and recorded. Deviations in gross motor development are frequently one of the earliest signs of such mental disorders as mental retardation (see Cognitive/Adaptive Skills cluster, p 61) or autistic disorder (see Social Interaction Behaviors cluster, p 277), and also such physical/neurosensory disorders as cerebral palsy or muscular dystrophy.

Normal variations in gross motor development are even more frequent. In fact, gross motor milestones exhibit the widest range of individual differences of any developmental domain. For example, the gross motor milestone "walking alone" can occur from 9 to 18 months and still be potentially a normal developmental variation. Fine motor development typically occurs within a much narrower range of normal variation. For example, the fine motor milestone, "neat pincer grasp," should consistently occur between 10 and 14 months of age.

Epidemiology

The prevalence of developmental coordination disorder is estimated to be as high as 6% for children between 5 and 11 years old.

DEVELOPMENTAL VARIATION	COMMON DEVELOPMENTAL PRESENTATIONS
V65.49 Developmental Coordination Variation These are normal variations in motor milestones that are typically encountered at all ages. They are based on a combination of intrinsic individual differences in neuromaturation and neurophysiology and extrinsic differences in experience.	**Infancy** The infant accomplishes milestones such as sitting, crawling, walking, "raking," or pincer grasp at the upper limits of normality for expected age. **Early Childhood** The child's gross or fine motor skills such as running, climbing, self-care, drawing, or onset of handedness are at the upper limits of normality for expected age. **Middle Childhood and Adolescence** The child's skills in such areas as printing, writing, physical, or athletic skills are less well developed but within the normal range.
	SPECIAL INFORMATION
	Developmental screening charts are a good source of normative information as to when 25%, 50%, 75%, and 90% of typical children perform various gross motor and fine motor milestones. Individual differences often "run in families," i.e., parents with a history of slow walking development are more likely to have children with a similar rate of development. Isolated delays of one or two skills beyond the normal range can occur but they should not cause any dysfunction in activities.

PROBLEM	COMMON DEVELOPMENTAL PRESENTATIONS
781.3 Developmental Coordination Problem Individual differences in motor development cause some impairment the further they deviate from the average by failing to meet parent or teacher expectations or unfavorable peer comparisons. Some refer to this problem as "late blooming."	**Infancy** The infant has late gross/fine motor milestones such as sitting, crawling, walking, "raking," or pincer grasp beyond normal expectations in more than two areas but not in most areas. **Early Childhood** The child has late gross/fine motor skills such as running, climbing, self-care, drawing, onset of handedness beyond normal expectations in more than two areas but not in most and it is sufficient to cause some impairment. **Middle Childhood and Adolescence** The child has late or problematic printing or writing (letter/word reversals) and physical/athletic skills ("last picked for any team").

	SPECIAL INFORMATION
	The further the acquisition of any specific motor skill deviates from the average, the more likely that it represents abnormal development. This is true for both the timing and quality of motor skills. Gross and fine motor skills should be assessed independently, since one may be atypical, delayed, or deviant while the other is in the normal range of developmental variation. Deprivation-induced motor symptoms may follow severe environmental deprivation or child abuse/neglect (see p 46). Motor development is generally the area of development most resistant to adverse parenting, so deprivation must be moderately severe to produce symptoms. The primary care physician faces the challenging task of differentiating a developmental variation in the quantity or quality of motor development from an actual mental or physical disorder. The much more common developmental variation requires parental reassurance and continued monitoring, whereas suspicions of a less common disorder require further diagnostic assessment. An intermediate category, problems in gross or fine motor development, is included to reflect the clinical reality of children in whom motor variations are sufficient to produce dysfunction and yet secondary symptoms do not fulfill the diagnostic criteria for an actual disorder. In many cases these problems in motor development, while diminishing in functional significance over time, persist into adulthood and constitute an area of development requiring compensatory skills and increased amounts of time and practice.

DISORDER	COMMON DEVELOPMENTAL PRESENTATIONS
315.4 Developmental Coordination Disorder Performance in daily activities that require motor coordination is substantially below that expected given the person's chronological age and measured intelligence. This may be manifest by marked delays in achieving motor milestones (e.g., walking, crawling, sitting), dropping things, "clumsiness," poor performance in sports, or poor handwriting. The disturbance significantly interferes with academic achievement or activities of daily living. The disturbance is not due to a general medical condition and does not meet criteria for an autistic disorder (see p 281). If mental retardation is present, the motor difficulties are in excess of those usually associated with it.	**Infancy** The infant has delayed gross or fine motor milestones well beyond reasonable allowance for individual differences in most cases. **Early Childhood** The child has delayed gross or fine motor skills (i.e., difficulty in holding a knife, buttoning clothes, running, playing ball games) in most areas. The child is markedly clumsy and can have motor planning problems. **Middle Childhood and Adolescence** The child has delayed development in most areas such as printing, writing, assembling puzzles, impairment in academic functions, building models, sporting activities that create significant impairment in academic and daily living functions.

SPECIAL INFORMATION

The degree of delay or deviation will aid in distinguishing a permanent disorder from a transient clinical problem. Additionally, the greater the number of specific item delays or deviations, the greater the likelihood that they indicate the presence of a mental or specific motor disorder or other health condition. The presence or absence of delays or deviations in other developmental domains (language, cognition, or social) will aid in identifying the specific type of disorder. If criteria are met for developmental coordination disorder and the symptoms cannot be attributed to a specific physical (general medical) condition or other mental disorder, the diagnosis should be developmental coordination disorder.

Physical and occupational therapists can provide more detailed information about the gross and fine motor functioning and can recommend programs. Other terms such as dyspraxia, remedial, and motor dysfunction may be used. Motor planning difficulties (the sequencing of movements) both fine and gross, may not be evident when observing the child doing what he or she chooses to do but will be seen when the child is asked to perform or imitate specific actions on demand.

DIFFERENTIAL DIAGNOSIS	SPECIAL INFORMATION
General Medical Conditions — Examples include: Cerebral palsy Muscular dystrophy Congenital hypotonia Progressive metabolic disorders Ataxia (post-varicella) Visual disorder Progressive lesions of the cerebellum	Deviation, or dissociations in motor development should preferentially alert the physician to the possibility of a chronic neurosensory condition or disorder. These are associated with abnormal neurological signs and tests. If signs and symptoms are nonprogressive (static), consider cerebral palsy. If evidence of neurological deterioration exists, consider muscular dystrophy or a progressive metabolic disorder. Developmental coordination disorder is not diagnosed if the symptoms are due to a general medical condition.

Substances — Examples include:
Prescription medications
  Anticonvulsants
  Neuroleptics (tardive dyskinesia)
Substances of abuse
  Alcohol
  Marijuana
  Cocaine
	Diagnosis is usually, but not always, temporally related. Tardive dyskinesia associated with neuroleptic use may vary in timing of onset.
	
	Consider prescription medications particularly in infants and young children, and substances of abuse particularly in older children and adolescents.

Mental Disorders **317,** Mental retardation **318.x,** **319** **299.00** Autistic disorder **314.xx** Attention-deficit/hyperactivity disorder	If mental retardation is present, the motor difficulties are in excess of those usually associated with that level of mental retardation to diagnose developmental coordination disorder.

COMMONLY COMORBID CONDITIONS	SPECIAL INFORMATION

Other Comorbid Mental Health Conditions — Examples include:
314.xx Attention-deficit/hyperactivity
         disorder
315.00 Reading disorder
315.1   Mathematics disorder
315.2   Disorder of written expression
315.39 Phonological disorder
315.31 Expressive language disorder
315.32 Mixed receptive-expressive
         language disorder
	Diagnosis is generally made at school age but may be made at younger ages, particularly in more severe cases. Developmental coordination disorder frequently occurs with ADHD and academic disorders.

Other General Medical Conditions — Examples include:
Chronic illness
  Anemia
  Endocrine
  Cardiac
  Pulmonary
  Renal
Obesity
Connective tissue disorders
	Developmental coordination can coexist with any other general medical condition. It should not be considered causal if the motor skills do not improve with improvement in the other conditions.

Presenting Complaints

not yet talking
does not speak clearly
mispronounces words
still talking baby talk
does not say enough
poorly understood by others
stutters

Definitions and Symptoms

Language development involves the acquisition of vocabulary and grammar as well as the principles that govern the use of this knowledge for social communication (pragmatics). Ordinarily, language is expressed through speech, which entails the organization and execution of coordinated movements of the vocal tract to produce a fluent and understandable (intelligible) utterance. Speech and language skills are critical for successful social and educational development. Furthermore, the successful development of speech and language depends on the integrity of many cognitive, auditory, and motor systems.

Individual differences in the rate of speech and language development can be substantial and yet still fall within the range of normal. This is most problematic for the clinician during the early stages of language development, occurring around 20 to 26 months of age. Most, if not all, children with language problems and disorders will have a delay in language development at this time. A large proportion of children with early delays, however, will later show normal language skills. Clinical action at this time should include an examination to rule out hearing loss and monitoring of development during the succeeding 6 to 12 months (or until about 3 years of age). If speech and language progress continues to be slow, or if there are other developmental concerns as well, refer the patient for further developmental examination. Clear identification of the nature and extent of speech and language skills requires assessment by a speech and language clinician. If questions of delay arise, it is better to err on the side of early evaluation by a speech and language clinician.

Epidemiology

Estimates suggest that 3% to 5% of children may be affected by the developmental type of expressive language disorder, and 3% of school-age children may be affected by mixed receptive-expressive language disorder. Approximately 2% to 3% of 6- to 7-year-olds present with moderate to severe phonological disorder, and 1% of prepubertal children are diagnosed with stuttering.

DEVELOPMENTAL VARIATION	COMMON DEVELOPMENTAL PRESENTATIONS
V65.49 Speech and Language Variation Language is acquired during early childhood in an ordered and systematic fashion with the child first learning to express isolated sounds, then phonemes, then words (generally starting with nouns and proceeding to verbs and then more complex grammatical terms). There is wide variation in the rate at which children acquire language — particularly at which they demonstrate expressive output. Children within the same family may develop their language patterns at different rates, especially when sisters and brother are compared.	**Infancy** The infant has differences from the norm in the development or amount of babbling, pointing, or onset of first words. Normal variance includes developmental malarticulation, normal shyness, and developmental dysfluencies. Syllabic or consonantal babbling is usually seen by about 10 months of age. Mild echolalia when the infant is at the one-word stage may be normal. The acquisition of single words can vary and not occur until 18 months while still being within the normal range. **Early Childhood** There is a wide range of normal variations in speech and language development. By the age of 2 years, the average child should be using about 50 or more words and combining words together into two-word (noun-verb) combinations. The typical 24-month-old can be understood by a stranger about 50% of the time, whereas the typical 36-month-old can be understood by a stranger about 75% of the time. Children from bilingual homes will develop both languages but may experience some delays. **Middle Childhood** The normal range of individual differences found in the speech and language skills of school age children is much smaller than that found during the preschool years. Children of this age should be fully intelligible and should be capable of engaging in basic conversational exchanges and regularly combining well-formed sentences into organized narrative discourse such as telling or retelling personal anecdotes and stories. Children may vary in their understanding of more subtle language forms including jokes, puns, etc. Normal variations are considerable with respect to the extent to which the child engages and is active in communicative interactions. **Adolescence** Communication skills at this age should approximate those expected of adults. Use of speaking styles that foster a feeling of identity with other members of this age group can be expected (e.g., interjections such as "like" or "you know" may be common).
	SPECIAL INFORMATION
	Concern by parents over instances of normal variation in the rate of language development, limited intelligibility, and occurrences of speech dysfluencies is common. Young children commonly use some idiosyncratic words ("bappy"). Receptive language may be more advanced than expressive language. Overgeneralization of grammatical rules ("she gived me the ball") is not uncommon. Speech dysfluencies that involve repetitions of whole words and phrases ("stuttering" or "stammering") are very common and usually transient. Consider as possible problems those delays outside the range described in the common developmental presentation. Communication development is often included in developmental inventories. There are also brief screening tools that focus on speech and language. Some authorities regard early speech and language screening as essential.

	SPECIAL INFORMATION, CONTINUED
	Differences in language development between children within the same family are not unusual and may be normal; however, when they are marked they may be a cue that there is a problem. There are also normal variations in the rate at which language develops in children. Other variations are social or cultural in origin, such as bilingualism or use of an ethnic or regional dialect. As such, assessment measures should be relevant for the cultural and linguistic group of the child. Children of some hearing-impaired parents (whether or not they are personally hearing impaired) may communicate in sign language instead of, or in addition to, speech. Severe environmental deprivation must also be distinguished.

PROBLEM	COMMON DEVELOPMENTAL PRESENTATIONS
V40.1 Speech and Language Problem Developmental speech and language problems arise when the delay or difference persists to a point that the child has a relative weakness in speech or language. These weaknesses may cause mild problems in young children but correct with minor interventions, or the children are able to compensate as they mature.	**Infancy** Early infant skills are similar to those found in normal developmental variation. Later behavior includes efforts to communicate through gesture accompanied by a lack in recognizable words. The infant has delay in comprehending the gestures, sounds, and words of others and using expressive language. **Early Childhood** The child has some difficulty comprehending age-appropriate conversation. The child communicates in a mildly less effective manner than appropriate for age with language delays characterized by immature sentence forms. The child's speech is generally understandable but contains some misarticulations and may have speech characterized by sound and symbol repetitions suggestive of stuttering. **Middle Childhood** The child has learning/language deficits, uses hyperverbal speech, uses speech that is fully understandable but contains errors involving 1 or 2 sounds such as "r" or "s." The child has speech dysfluencies similar to those of early childhood suggestive of stuttering but continues to have few, if any, sound prolongations or grimaces in a waxing-waning pattern. The child has weak conversational skills or constructs short narratives with limited collusion or organizational structure. In middle childhood, language delays should no longer be obvious, although some limitations in language facility may be present and may restrict school performance. **Adolescence** The adolescent has minor dysfluencies not impairing intelligibility or has a relative weakness in expressive or receptive language.
	SPECIAL INFORMATION
	Otitis media or other types of conductive or sensory neural hearing loss should be considered. The communication problems in this section are likely to follow a developmental course, with misarticulations and limited vocabulary being the most obvious problems in early childhood, minor misarticulations, sentence structure problems in late, early, and middle childhood, and conversation and narrative problems in middle childhood and adolescence, with the degree of deviation from normal expectations diminishing with age. Most of these conditions warrant referral for a speech-language evaluation and consideration of clinical management programs. In the case of stuttering, refer the child for evaluation if the dysfluency persists for longer than 6 to 8 weeks. Approximately 80% of children with stuttering recover, with up to 60% recovering spontaneously before age 16 years.

DISORDER	COMMON DEVELOPMENTAL PRESENTATIONS

315.31 Expressive Language Disorder

The scores obtained from standardized individually administered measures of expressive language development are substantially below those obtained from standardized measures of both nonverbal intellectual capacity and receptive language development. The disturbance may be manifest clinically by symptoms that include having a markedly limited vocabulary, making errors in tense, or having difficulty in recalling words or producing sentences with developmentally appropriate length or complexity.

The difficulties with expressive language interfere with academic or occupational achievement or with social communication.

Does not meet criteria for mixed receptive-expressive language disorder, or a pervasive developmental disorder. Expressive language disorder can be diagnosed in the presence of mental retardation, a speech-motor or sensory deficit, or environmental deprivation but only if the language difficulties are in excess of language problems usually associated with these problems.

315.32 Mixed Receptive-Expressive Language Disorder

The scores obtained from a battery of standardized individually administered measures of both receptive and expressive language development are substantially below those obtained from standardized measures of nonverbal intellectual capacity. Symptoms include those for expressive language disorder as well as difficulty understanding words, sentences, or specific types of words, such as spatial terms.

The difficulties with receptive and expressive language significantly interfere with academic or occupational achievement or with social communication. Mixed receptive-expressive language disorder is distinguished from expressive language disorder by the presence in the former of significant impairment in receptive language. The same exclusions apply to both expressive language disorder and mixed-receptive language disorder.

307.9 Communication Disorder, NOS

Infancy
During the first years of life, the child's communication does not develop into using a series of gestures and words together to indicate the child's needs and desires.

Early Childhood
The child with an expressive language disorder has expressive language delay, is unable to use language as part of pretend play, is unable to communicate, and has very limited speech, most of which is unintelligible. The child with a mixed disorder in addition has limited vocabulary, has immature sentence structure that often lacks certain grammatical markers, has very limited communication capacities, has socially inappropriate communication, uses hyperverbal or "cocktail party" speech in which the child talks too much or in a disinhibited way. The child demonstrates an impairment in receptive language development (e.g., difficulty understanding words, sentences, or specific types of words).

Middle Childhood
Symptoms are similar to those of early childhood but the skills are more sophisticated. The child cannot organize sentences into a conversational exchange or narrative discourses.

Adolescence
The adolescent has the same symptoms as those in middle childhood, shows continued signs of difficulty with several speech sounds, particularly in longer words, has limited vocabulary as well as continued grammatical errors, poor conversation, or narrative discourse.

SPECIAL INFORMATION

These developmental speech and language disorders often occur together so that speech sound production difficulties and language delay coincide. Also, these disorders are often associated with other developmental disorders such as mental retardation or learning disorders. Children with forms of pervasive developmental disorder may also engage in communicative efforts that are socially inappropriate. Those with severe language disorder may have selective mutism. Speech is marked by numerous speech sound errors and thus is difficult to understand. Developmental speech and language disorders result in restrictions in the child's ability to meet the functional demands of communication. Thus, the child is limited in his or her ability to understand and express those things that are needed for the activities of daily living. Approximately half of the children with expressive language disorder appear to outgrow it; half appear to have more long-lasting difficulties. Persistent delays in speech and language development may be indicators of hearing impairment, mental retardation (see Cognitive/Adaptive Skills cluster, p 61), or autistic disorder (see Social Interaction Behaviors cluster, p 277), and may also place the child at risk for later reading problems (see Academic Skills cluster, p 69).

Language disorders may be either acquired or developmental. In the acquired type, impairment presents after a period of normal development as a result of a neurological or other general medical condition (e.g., encephalitis, head trauma, irradiation). In the developmental type, an impairment in language exists that is not associated with a neurological insult of known origin and is characterized by a slow rate of language development in which speech may begin late and advance slowly.

DISORDER	COMMON DEVELOPMENTAL PRESENTATIONS
307.0 Stuttering Disturbance in the normal fluency and time patterning of speech (inappropriate for the individual's age), characterized by frequent occurrences of one or more of the following: sound and syllable repetitions, sound prolongations, interjections, broken words (pauses within a word), audible or silent blocking (filled or unfilled pauses in speech), word substitutions to avoid problematic words, words pronounced with an excess of physical tension, monosyllabic whole-word repetitions. The disturbance in fluency interferes with academic or occupational achievement or with social communication. **315.39 Phonological Disorder** Failure to use developmentally expected speech sounds that are appropriate for age and dialect (e.g., errors in sound production use, representation, or organization such as, but not limited to, substitutions of one sound for another [use of "t" for target "k" sound] or omissions of sounds as final consonants). The difficulties in speech sound production interfere with academic or occupational achievement or with social communication. If mental retardation, a speech-motor or sensory deficit, or environmental deprivation is present, the speech difficulties are in excess of those usually associated with these problems.	**Infancy** Not relevant at this age. **Early Childhood** The child stutters with frequent (10% or more of words produced) repetitions of sounds, syllables, or short words, as well as sound prolongations and blockages. The child may produce unintelligible speech. **Middle Childhood** The child stutters with similar signs as those described in early childhood. The child produces articulation errors, fails to form speech sounds correctly, exhibits a deficit in linguistic categorization of speech sounds, unintelligible speech, sound omissions, and substitutions. Lisping is particularly common and the child may misorder sounds within syllables and words (e.g., "aks" for "ask"). **Adolescence** The adolescent stutters with similar signs as those described in early childhood. The adolescent fails to produce age-appropriate speech sounds as in middle childhood.

SPECIAL INFORMATION
A family history of stuttering may be more likely in instances of persistent stuttering. In middle childhood, stuttering is likely to worsen when the child is anxious or under stress. The child may have frequent associated behaviors such as eye blinking and twitching. Stuttering often is more severe when there is special pressure to communicate (e.g., giving a report at school). Stuttering may be absent during oral reading, singing, or talking to inanimate objects or to pets.

DIFFERENTIAL DIAGNOSIS	SPECIAL INFORMATION
General Medical Conditions— Examples include: Hearing impairment Neuromotor impairment Genetic disorders or syndromes impairing cognitive/adaptive abilities Motor impairment Recurrent otitis media with intermittent hearing loss Dysarthria Moebius syndrome	
Substances None	
Mental Disorders 313.23 Selective mutism 317, Mental retardation 318.x, 319 299.00 Autistic disorder	Learning disability is a school age diagnosis.

COMMONLY COMORBID CONDITIONS	SPECIAL INFORMATION
Other Comorbid Mental Health Conditions — Examples include: 315.1 Mathematics disorder 314.xx Attention-deficit/hyperactivity disorder 307.6 Enuresis 315.4 Developmental coordination disorder 315.00 Reading disorder 315.2 Disorder of written expression 317, Mental retardation 318.x, 319	Attention-deficit/hyperactivity disorder (see Hyperactive/Impulsive Behaviors cluster, p 93) is not often diagnosed until school age. Additional difficulties may include motor articulation problems, phonological errors, slow speech, syllable repetitions, monotonous intonation, and stress patterns. Mental retardation may also be coded only when the extent of the language difficulties goes beyond what would be expected with that level of mental retardation.
Other General Medical Conditions — Examples include: Aphasia Dysarthria Apraxia Agnosia Cerebral palsy Cleft lip/palate Hydrocephalus/spina bifida Acquired aphasia (Landau-Kleffner syndrome)	

Impulsive/Hyperactive or Inattentive Behaviors

Hyperactive/Impulsive Behaviors

Inattentive Behaviors

Presenting Complaints

can't sit still
restless and fidgety
talks constantly
interrupts
acts without thinking

Definition and Symptoms

Activity includes any kind of motor activity ranging from gross motor movement to fidgeting with hands and feet and excessive talking. Impulsive behaviors are actions done quickly without thought of the consequences. Motor activity, including thoughtless motor behaviors, is a part of normal human behavior and ranges from sluggish, overly careful behavior to constant motion with total disregard for the effects of the behavior on others.

Motor activity is normally in the high range in early childhood development until early gross motor skills are consolidated (ages 2 to 3 years). Normally high activity levels and impulsive tendencies continue until early adolescence, although they are gradually reduced. Impulsive behaviors reduce considerably as children enter the piagetian stage of concrete operations (i.e., when 7 to 11 years old), when causal connections are more clearly understood.

Excessive activity and impulsivity are detected only by observations of the child in multiple settings over time. Judgments about the degree of behavioral deviation are based mainly on the effect of the behaviors on other people and on the child's ability to accomplish age-appropriate tasks such as learning in school. Excessive levels of activity and impulsivity are seen in attention-deficit/hyperactivity disorder (ADHD) and in anxiety and mood disorders. It can also be seen in other more severe conditions such as pervasive developmental disorder or schizophrenia but rarely as an isolated or predominant symptom. There are three subtypes of ADHD including attention-deficit/hyperactivity disorder, combined type; attention-deficit/hyperactivity disorder, predominantly inattentive type; and attention-deficit/hyperactivity disorder, predominantly hyperactive-impulsive type.

Epidemiology

The prevalence of ADHD is estimated at 3% to 5% in school-age children. With the new *DSM-IV* criteria the preliminary studies suggest that the rates are increased due to the definition of the three subtypes. This is essentially accounted for by the inclusion of primarily inattentive and hyperactive/impulsive subtypes. Higher levels of activity and impulsivity are seen in young children (approximately 3 to 10 years of age), especially in boys. The activity level normally decreases noticeably during adolescence. The disorder is much more frequent in males than in females, with male-to-female ratios ranging from 4:1 to 9:1 depending on the setting.

Etiology

There is a higher frequency of ADHD in first-degree relatives, suggesting a genetic component. ADHD also may be associated with a history of child abuse and neglect (see p 45), multiple foster placements (see p 45), neurotoxin exposure (e.g., lead poisoning), infections (e.g., encephalitis), drug exposure in utero, low birth weight, and mental retardation.

DEVELOPMENTAL VARIATION	COMMON DEVELOPMENTAL PRESENTATIONS
V65.49 Hyperactive/Impulsive Variation Young children in infancy and in the preschool years are normally very active and impulsive and may need constant supervision to avoid injury. Their constant activity may be stressful to adults who do not have the energy or patience to tolerate the behavior. During school years and adolescence, activity may be high in play situations and impulsive behaviors may normally occur, especially in peer pressure situations. High levels of hyperactive/impulsive behavior do not indicate a problem or disorder if the behavior does not impair function.	**Infancy** Infants will vary in their responses to stimulation. Some infants may be overactive to sensations such as touch and sound and may squirm away from the caregiver, while others find it pleasurable to respond with increased activity. **Early Childhood** The child runs in circles, doesn't stop to rest, may bang into objects or people, and asks questions constantly. **Middle Childhood** The child plays active games for long periods. The child may occasionally do things impulsively, particularly when excited. **Adolescence** The adolescent engages in active social activities (e.g., dancing) for long periods, may engage in risky behaviors with peers.
	SPECIAL INFORMATION
	Activity should be thought of not only in terms of actual movement, but also in terms of variations in responding to touch, pressure, sound, light, and other sensations. Also, for the infant and young child, activity and attention are related to the interaction between the child and the caregiver, e.g., when sharing attention and playing together. Activity and impulsivity often normally increase when the child is tired or hungry and decrease when sources of fatigue or hunger are addressed. Activity normally may increase in new situations or when the child may be anxious. Familiarity then reduces activity. Both activity and impulsivity must be judged in the context of the caregiver's expectations and the level of stress experienced by the caregiver. When expectations are unreasonable, the stress level is high, and/or the parent has an emotional disorder (especially depression [see p 46, emotional disorder of parent V61.9]), the adult may exaggerate the child's level of activity/impulsivity. Activity level is a variable of temperament (see Children's Responses to Environmental Situations and Potentially Stressful Events Preamble, p 31). The activity level of some children is on the high end of normal from birth and continues to be high throughout their development.

PROBLEM	COMMON DEVELOPMENTAL PRESENTATIONS
V40.3 Hyperactive/Impulsive Behavior Problem These behaviors become a problem when they are intense enough to begin to disrupt relationships with others or begin to affect the acquisition of age-appropriate skills. The child displays some of the symptoms listed on p 00 for the ADHD predominantly hyperactive/impulsive subtype. However, the behaviors are not sufficiently intense to qualify for a behavioral disorder such as ADHD, or of a mood disorder (see Sadness and Related Symptoms cluster, p 153), or anxiety disorder (see Anxious Symptoms cluster, p 145). A problem degree of this behavior is also likely to be accompanied by other behaviors such as negative emotional behaviors or aggressive/oppositional behaviors.	**Infancy** The infant squirms and has early motor development with increased climbing. Sensory underreactivity and overreactivity as described in developmental variations can be associated with high activity levels. **Early Childhood** The child frequently runs into people or knocks things down during play, gets injured frequently, and does not want to sit for stories or games. **Middle Childhood** The child may butt into other children's games, interrupts frequently, and has problems completing chores. **Adolescence** The adolescent engages in "fooling around" that begins to annoy others and fidgets in class or while watching television.
	SPECIAL INFORMATION
	In infancy and early childhood, a problem level of these behaviors may be easily confused with cognitive problems such as limited intelligence or specific developmental problems (see Cognitive/Adaptive Skills cluster, p 61 and Speech and Language cluster, p 83). However, cognitive problems and hyperactive/impulsive symptoms can occur simultaneously. A problem level of these behaviors may also be seen from early childhood on, as a response to neglect (see p 46), physical/sexual abuse (see p 45), or other chronic stress, and this possibility should be considered.

DISORDER	COMMON DEVELOPMENTAL PRESENTATIONS

Attention-Deficit/Hyperactivity Disorder

314.01 Predominantly Hyperactive-Impulsive Type

This subtype should be used if six (or more) of the following symptoms of hyper-activity-impulsivity (but fewer than six symptoms of inattention [see p 103]) have persisted for at least 6 months. They present before the age of 7 years. The symptoms need to be present to a significantly greater degree than is appropriate for the age, cognitive ability, and gender of the child, and the symptoms should be present in more than one setting (e.g., school and home).

Hyperactive-impulsive symptoms:

These symptoms must be present to a degree that is maladaptive and inconsistent with developmental level, resulting in significant impairment.

Hyperactivity
- often fidgets with hands/feet or squirms in seat
- often leaves seat in classroom or in other situations in which remaining seated is expected
- often runs about or climbs excessively in situation in which it is inappropriate (in adolescents or adults, may be limited to subjective feelings of restlessness)
- often has difficulty playing or engaging in leisure activities quietly
- is often "on the go" or often acts as if "driven by a motor"
- often talks excessively

Impulsivity
- often blurts out answers before questions are completed
- often has difficulty awaiting turn
- often interrupts or intrudes on others

(For criteria for inattention symptoms, see Inattentive Behaviors cluster, p 103.)

Infancy
The infant squirms frequently and has early motor development with excessive climbing. The infant has a hard time focusing on people or objects and squirms constantly. The infant does not organize purposeful gestures or behavior. The infant may show interest in gross motor activities such as excessive climbing but may also have difficulties in motor planning and sequencing (imitating complex movements). However, these behaviors are nonspecific and a disorder diagnosis is extremely difficult to make in this age group.

Early Childhood
The child runs through the house, jumps and climbs excessively on furniture, will not sit still to eat or be read to, and is often into things.

Middle Childhood
The child is often talking and interrupting, cannot sit still at mealtimes, is often fidgeting when watching television, makes noise that is disruptive, and grabs from others.

Adolescence
The adolescent is restless and fidgety while doing any and all quiet activities, interrupts and "bugs" other people, and gets into trouble frequently. Hyperactive symptoms decrease or are replaced with a sense of restlessness.

SPECIAL INFORMATION

Specific environmental situations and stressors often make a significant contribution to the severity of these behaviors, though they are seldom entirely responsible for a disorder-level diagnosis of these behaviors. Situations and stressors that should be systematically assessed include:

Marital discord/divorce, p 44
Physical abuse/sexual abuse, p 45
Mental disorder of parent, p 46
Other family relationship problems, p 45

Difficulties with cognitive/adaptive skills, academic skills, and speech and language skills often lead to frustration and low self-esteem that contribute to the severity of these behaviors. These conditions may also co-exist with ADHD and therefore should be systematically assessed.

DISORDER, CONTINUED	COMMON DEVELOPMENTAL PRESENTATIONS, CONTINUED

314.01 Predominantly Hyperactive-Impulsive Type, continued

Some hyperactive-impulsive or inattentive symptoms that caused impairment were present before age 7 years. Some impairment from the symptoms is present in two or more settings (e.g., at school and at home). There must be clear evidence of clinically significant impairment in social, academic, or occupational functioning. The symptoms do not occur exclusively during the course of an autistic disorder (see following differential diagnostic information), and are not better accounted for by another mental disorder (see following differential diagnosis information).

314.01 Combined Type

This subtype should be used if criteria, six (or more) symptoms of hyperactivity-impulsivity and six (or more) of the symptoms of the inattention (see p 107), have persisted for at least 6 months.

314.9 Attention-Deficit/ Hyperactivity Disorder, NOS

(see *DSM-IV* Criteria Appendix, p 316)

SPECIAL INFORMATION

Specific environmental situations and stressors often make a significant contribution to the severity of these behaviors, though they are seldom entirely responsible for a disorder-level diagnosis of these behaviors. Situations and stressors that should be systematically assessed include:

Marital discord/divorce, p **44**
Physical abuse/sexual abuse, p **45**
Mental disorder of parent, p **46**
Other family relationship problems, p **45**
Loss/bereavement, p **43**

Difficulties with cognitive/adaptive skills, academic skills, and speech and language skills often lead to frustration and low self-esteem that both contribute to the severity of these behaviors. These conditions may also co-exist with ADHD and therefore should be systematically assessed.

DIFFERENTIAL DIAGNOSIS	SPECIAL INFORMATION
General Medical Conditions—Examples include: Any disease that acutely affects central nervous system (CNS) function may produce symptoms of hyperactivity/impulsivity. In order to establish a causal connection, there must be a behavioral change seen *following* the onset of the central nervous system disease. Examples include: Meningitis Encephalitis Head injury CNS tumor Cerebral vascular accident Lupus, with CNS inflammation CNS chemotherapy Iron-deficiency anemia Lead poisoning However, most disorders affecting CNS function cannot be clearly associated with a change in behavior. Since the treatment of the ADHD behaviors is the same whether or not there is an associated neurologic disorder, it is accepted to consider these disorders as comorbid conditions (see below). Any chronic medical condition that increases anxiety or depression may result in hyperactive/impulsive behaviors. Examples include: Insulin-dependent diabetes Serious physical injury with loss of function Chronic renal disease Neoplastic disease requiring chemotherapy	Both the medical and mental conditions can be coded. Treatment of the health condition should ameliorate the symptoms of the behavior problem/disorder. Visual and hearing impairments in infants should be ruled out.

DIFFERENTIAL DIAGNOSIS, CONTINUED	SPECIAL INFORMATION, CONTINUED
Substances Any medication that affects CNS functioning or produces anxiety or depression may result in behavioral symptoms of hyperactivity/impulsivity. Examples include: Theophylline Antihistamines Phenobarbital Systemic steroids Substances that are stimulants may produce symptoms of hyperactivity-impulsivity. Examples include: Cocaine Phencyclidine Stimulants, e.g., amphetamines	Code the substance use only. **292.89** Other Substance Intoxication **292.0** Other Substance Withdrawal Removal of the substance should ameliorate the behavioral symptoms, thus confirming the casual connections.
Mental Disorders Some mental disorders often include hyperactive/impulsive behaviors as part of their presentation. When the symptoms of these disorders are the initial and primary presentation, the hyperactive/impulsive behaviors should be considered secondary if the symptoms were not independent of the other disorder. Examples include: **299.0** Autistic disorder **296.xx** Major depressive disorder **300.02** Generalized anxiety disorder **300.01** Panic disorder **309.81** Posttraumatic stress disorder **301.82** Avoidant personality disorder **300.4** Dysthymic disorder **309.21** Separation anxiety disorder **300.23** Social phobia	Code only the mental disorder. In the case of these mental disorders, treatment of the disorder should ameliorate the hyperactive/impulsive behaviors, thus establishing the causal relationship. If the child with autistic disorder manifests significant hyperactive/impulsive behavior that warrants a focus of treatment, code both autism and hyperactive/impulsive behaviors problem or disorder (ADHD).

COMMONLY COMORBID CONDITIONS	SPECIAL INFORMATION
Other Comorbid Mental Health Conditions If hyperactive/impulsive behaviors are associated with significant underachievement in academic or motor skills, consider: **315.00** Reading disorder **315.1** Mathematics disorder **315.2** Disorder of written expression **315.4** Developmental coordination disorder **315.xx,** Communication disorders **307.xx** If hyperactive/impulsive behaviors are associated with chronic motor and vocal tics, consider: **307.23** Tourette's disorder If hyperactive/impulsive behaviors are associated with significantly subaverage general intellectual functioning and by significant limitation in adaptive functioning, consider: **317** Mild mental retardation **318.0** Moderate mental retardation **319** Mental retardation, severity unspecified If hyperactive/impulsive behaviors are associated with significant oppositional and defiant behavior, consider: **313.81** Oppositional defiant disorder If hyperactive/impulsive behaviors are associated with significant antisocial behaviors, consider: **312.81** Conduct disorder childhood onset **312.82** Conduct disorder adolescent onset	Code both the hyperactive/impulsive problem or disorder (ADHD) and the academic, motor skills, or communication disorder. Tic disorders frequently occur with ADHD. Stimulant medications can exacerbate tics so careful assessment and consultation with a specialist may be required. For mild or moderate mental retardation, code both the mental retardation and the hyperactive/impulsive behavior problem or disorder (ADHD). For severe levels of mental retardation, code only the mental retardation, even if behavior problems typical of ADHD are present. Code both conditions. Code both conditions.

COMMONLY COMORBID CONDITIONS, CONTINUED	SPECIAL INFORMATION, CONTINUED
Other Comorbid Mental Health Conditions, continued The same disorders that were present in the differential diagnoses may also occur simultaneously. If hyperactive/impulsive behaviors have been accompanied since the time of their initial appearance with symptoms of dysthymic disorder, symptoms of major depression, or symptoms of an anxiety disorder, consider: **300.4** Dysthymic disorder **296.xx** Major depressive disorder **300.02** Generalized anxiety disorder **309.21** Separation anxiety disorder **301.82** Avoidant personality disorder **309.81** Posttraumatic stress disorder **300.23** Social phobia	Code both (or more) conditions.
Other General Medical Conditions Any general medical condition affecting CNS functioning may coexist with hyperactive/impulsive behavior problem or disorder (ADHD). Examples include: Seizure disorder Fetal alcohol syndrome Prematurity Anoxic brain damage Perinatal substance abuse Neurocutaneous syndrome Post-brain injury syndrome Post-meningitic syndrome Thyroid problems	Code both conditions.

Definitions and Symptoms

The inability to attend to any activity or object for any appreciable length of time indicates inattentive behaviors. The child's attention, therefore, quickly wanders from one thing to another. The rapid shifts in attention are often accompanied by a failure to attend to or perceive details, and thus the child may miss many subtle aspects of an object or situation. The child is unable to bring an activity to its natural and expected conclusion. This includes active pursuits such as playing a game or drawing a picture, and passive activities such as listening to a story. The lack of persistence is not related to frustration because of an inability to perform a particular task, but is more related to the child's marked distractibility.

The attention span of children normally increases with age, so that inattention must be evaluated in the context of the child's age and developmental stage. The degree of persistence that is normal for a child will vary with age, with younger children being able to persist in a given activity for much shorter periods of time than older children.

Epidemiology

The prevalence of attention-deficit/hyperactivity disorder is estimated at 3% to 5% in school-age children. With the new *DSM-IV* criteria, preliminary studies suggest the rates may be higher because they now include all three subtypes. Data on prevalence in adolescence and adulthood are limited. The disorder is much more frequent in males than in females, with male-to-female ratios ranging from 4:1 to 9:1 depending on the setting. Preliminary studies of the *DSM-IV* subtypes suggest that the predominances of males is lower (2:1) for the predominantly inattentive subtype.

Etiology

Attention span is one aspect of temperament and varies normally along a wide range based on genetic factors. Many of the attention problems or disorders are thought to have a genetic component because of the high frequency in first-degree relatives. In addition, the attention problems or disorders can be associated with disorders of or damage to central nervous system function. A short attention span and easy distractibility are associated with all types of disturbance in development, ranging from delays in speech and language skills to delays in cognitive/adaptive skills (see Cognitive/Adaptive Skills cluster, p 61, and Speech and Language cluster, p 83). In addition, problems with attention frequently accompany symptoms of anxiety or mood problems.

Environmental stresses of all kinds also affect attention span. Abuse (see p 45) or neglect should be considered, particularly in a child with attention problems. Any child who is hungry, tired, or uncomfortable will often be inattentive.

DEVELOPMENTAL VARIATION	COMMON DEVELOPMENTAL PRESENTATIONS
V65.49 Inattention Variation A young child will have a short attention span that will increase as the child matures. The inattention should be appropriate for the child's level of development and not cause any impairment.	**Infancy** Attention varies depending on the saliency of the stimulus and the individual differences in the infant's ability to process auditory, visual, or motor patterns. One child may fix on a parent's voice, while another will respond to animated facial expression. **Early Childhood** The preschooler has difficulty attending, except briefly, to a story book or a quiet task such as coloring or drawing. **Middle Childhood** The child may not persist very long with a task the child does not want to do such as read an assigned book, homework, or a task that requires concentration such as cleaning something. **Adolescence** The adolescent is easily distracted from tasks he or she does not desire to perform.

SPECIAL INFORMATION
Infants and preschoolers usually have very short attention spans and normally do not persist with activities for long, so that diagnosing this problem in younger children may be difficult. Some parents may have a low tolerance for developmentally appropriate inattention. Although watching television cartoons for long periods of time appears to reflect a long attention span, it does not reflect longer attention spans because most television segments require short (2- to 3-minute) attention spans and they are very stimulating. Normally, attention span varies greatly depending upon the child's or adolescent's interest and skill in the activity, so much so that a short attention span for a particular task may reflect the child's skill or interest in that task.

PROBLEM	COMMON DEVELOPMENTAL PRESENTATIONS
V40.3 Inattention Problem A problem exists when some of the symptoms, listed on the next page for the ADHD predominantly inattentive type are present and they create some difficulties for the child's parents and teachers and begin to affect some areas of academic and social functioning. However, the behaviors are not sufficiently intense to qualify for a behavioral disorder.	**Infancy** The infant does not show significant progress in attending to caregiver's face or an age-appropriate toy — i.e., infant does not increase attention from 5 to 10 seconds during first months to a few minutes at the end of the first year. The infant is unable to complete even short tasks: crawling to objects, playing peek-a-boo, or placing even one or two blocks in a box. The infant lacks persistence when eating — a bite of food is taken but really not finished before interest is expressed in something else on the table or in an activity not related to eating. **Early Childhood** The child is sometimes unable to complete games or activities without being distracted, is unable to complete a game with another child of comparable age, and only attends to any activity for a very short period of time before shifting attention to another object or activity. Symptoms are present to the degree that they cause some family difficulties. **Middle Childhood and Adolescence** At times the child misses some instructions and explanations in school, begins a number of activities without completing them, has some difficulties completing games with other children or grownups, becomes distracted, tends to give up easily, may not complete or succeed at new activities, has some social deficiency, and does not pick up subtle social cues from others. See the symptom list for the ADHD predominantly inattentive subtype on the next page.

SPECIAL INFORMATION
Motor planning, such as the ability to do a puzzle or making a toy work, should not be confused with an attention problem. Consider chaotic family situation — marital discord, separation, divorce (see p 44), or depression (see p 46), and physical and/or sexual abuse or neglect (see p 45).

DISORDER	COMMON DEVELOPMENTAL PRESENTATIONS
Attention-Deficit/Hyperactivity Disorder: **314.00 Predominantly Inattentive Type** This subtype should be used if six (or more) of the following symptoms of inattention (but fewer than six symptoms of hyperactivity/impulsivity [see p 93]) have persisted for at least 6 months. *Inattention* These symptoms must be present to a degree that is maladaptive and inconsistent with developmental level. • often fails to give close attention to details, makes careless mistakes in schoolwork or other activities • often has difficulty sustaining attention in tasks or play activities • often does not seem to listen when spoken to directly • often does not follow through on instructions and fails to finish schoolwork or chores (not due to oppositional behavior or failure to understand instructions) • often has difficulty organizing tasks and activities • often avoids, dislikes, or is reluctant to engage in tasks that require sustained mental effort (such as schoolwork or homework) • often loses things necessary for tasks or activities (e.g., toys, school assignments, pencils, books, tools) • is often easily distracted by extraneous stimuli • is often forgetful in daily activities (For criteria for hyperactive/impulsive symptoms, see Hyperactive/Impulsive Behaviors cluster, p 93.)	**Infancy** The infant evidences only fleeting attention (in and out) and is unable to focus for more than 5 to 6 seconds on a caregiver's facial expressions, presentation of a toy, or other interactive opportunity. Initially, attempts to increase attention require tremendous effort on the part of the caregiver, such as holding a toy for the infant to reach for. However, these behaviors are nonspecific and a disorder diagnosis is extremely difficult to make in this age group. **Early Childhood** The child is unable to function and play appropriately, and may appear immature, does not engage in any activity long enough, is easily distracted, is unable to complete activities, has a much shorter attention span than other children the same age, often misses important aspects of an object or situation (e.g., rules of games or sequences), and does not persist in various self-care tasks (dressing or washing) to the same extent as other children of comparable age. The child shows problems in many settings over a long period of time and is affected functionally. **Middle Childhood and Adolescence** The child has significant school and social problems, often shifts activities, does not complete tasks, is messy and careless about schoolwork, starts tasks prematurely and without appropriate review of the instructions, appears as if his or her mind is elsewhere and as if he or she were not listening, has difficulty organizing tasks, dislikes activities that require close concentration, is easily distracted, and is often forgetful.

DISORDER, CONTINUED	SPECIAL INFORMATION, CONTINUED
314.01 Combined Type If criteria are met for both inattention and hyperactivity/impulsivity, then code combined type. This subtype should be used if criteria, six (or more) of the symptoms of hyperactivity/impulsivity (see p 97) and six (or more) symptoms of inattention (see p 107), have persisted for at least 6 months. Some inattention or inattentive symptoms that caused impairment were present before age 7 years. Some impairment from the symptoms is present in two or more settings (e.g., at school and at home). There must be clear evidence of clinically significant impairment in social, academic, or occupational functioning. The symptoms do not occur exclusively during the course of an autistic disorder (see following differential diagnostic information), and are not better accounted for by another mental disorder (see following differential diagnosis information). **314.9 Attention-Deficit/ Hyperactivity Disorder, NOS** (see *DSM-IV* Criteria Appendix, p 316)	Consider chaotic family situation — marital discord (see p 44) or parental depression (see p 46), and physical and/or sexual abuse or neglect (see p 45).

DIFFERENTIAL DIAGNOSIS	SPECIAL INFORMATION
General Medical Conditions Any condition that affects central nervous system function may result in inattention. Examples include: Seizure disorder, particularly petit mal Meningitis Encephalitis Brain injury Systemic lupus Thyroid disorder Iron-deficiency anemia Fragile X syndrome Fetal alcohol syndrome	Only when problems with attention first appear in the context of one of these medical conditions and resolve with the correction of the condition should the medical conditions be considered causal differential diagnosis. In this situation, code only the medical condition. The attention problem should decrease when the medical condition is treated or abates.
Substances Many substances may cause inattention problems while they are being used. Examples include: Cocaine Amphetamines Marijuana Phencyclidine Many medications that affect central nervous system function may result in inattention. Examples include: Antihistamines Neuroleptics Thyroid medications Phenobarbital	Only when the substance or medication use is followed by the problems with attention should the relationship be considered causal. Discontinuance of the substance or medication should alleviate the attention problem. Code only the substance or medication use.
Mental Disorders Several mental disorders other than attention-deficit/hyperactivity disorder include inattention as one of their symptoms. When the inattention symptoms are best considered part of the other disorder, that disorder is part of the differential diagnosis of inattentive behaviors. Examples include: **299.00** Autistic disorder **309.81** Posttraumatic stress disorder **300.01** Panic disorder **296.xx** Major depressive disorder	Code only the mental disorder. Treatment of the mental disorder should alleviate the inattention symptoms.

COMMONLY COMORBID CONDITIONS	SPECIAL INFORMATION
Other Comorbid Mental Health Conditions — Mental Disorders A number of behavioral syndromes labeled as mental health problems or disorders occur in children who also have attention deficit problems or disorders. Both conditions (or more) have been present usually since early childhood. Examples include: **313.81** Oppositional defiant disorder **312.81** Conduct disorder childhood onset **312.82** Conduct disorder adolescent onset **315.39** Phonological disorder **307.0** Stuttering **315.00** Reading disorder **315.1** Mathematics disorder **315.2** Disorder of written expression **315.31** Expressive language disorder **315.32** Mixed receptive-expressive language disorder **317, 318.x, 319** Mental retardation, mild and moderate **300.02** Generalized anxiety disorder **300.4** Dysthymic disorder **307.23** Tourette's disorder	Code both conditions as appropriate. For mild or moderate mental retardation, code both the mental retardation and the inattention behavior problem or disorder (ADHD). For severe and profound levels of mental retardation, code only the mental retardation, even if behavior problems typical of ADHD are present.
Other General Medical Conditions — Examples include: Seizure disorder, particularly petit mal Meningitis Encephalitis Brain injury Systemic lupus Thyroid disorder Iron-deficiency anemia Fragile X syndrome Fetal alcohol syndrome	Chronic illness, pain, and discomfort may affect attention span. Chronic infections or malnutrition may affect a child's ability to persist in activities. These conditions will only rarely lead to a diagnosis of ADHD. If the general medical condition produces only temporary inattentiveness, code as in differentiated diagnosis (above).

Negative/Antisocial Behaviors

Negative Emotional Behaviors

Aggressive/Oppositional Behaviors

Secretive Antisocial Behaviors

> **Presenting Complaints**
>
> crying and whining
> yelling and cursing
> temper tantrums
> angry outbursts

Definitions and Symptoms

Negative emotional behaviors are physical and verbal manifestations of negative emotions including anger, frustration, and irritation. These behaviors range from mild forms such as facial grimacing and whining to severe forms such as temper tantrums or yelling and cursing. In general, the severity of the behavior is directly related to the strength of the negative emotion. These behaviors, even when they are of normal intensity and frequency, may be a problem for caregivers who have difficulty responding to negative emotions and behaviors. Adults who are depressed (see mental disorder of parent, p 46) or under significant stress are particularly sensitive to these behaviors.

Assessment of the severity of these behaviors should involve observations over time and in many different situations, since brief outbursts of negative emotional behaviors are common and normal. When the behaviors are more frequent and intense than normal and when they persist beyond the specific developmental periods with which such behaviors are commonly associated, they become problems. When they are also associated with other symptoms, such as those of depression (see Sadness and Related Symptoms cluster, p 153), they may be manifestations of a mood disorder. The evaluation of severity must take into account the characteristics of the caregiver or reporter whose observations may be biased or whose behavior may be provoking the negative emotional behaviors in the child. The evaluation of severity also depends on the effects of this behavior on peers and caregivers. When negative emotional behaviors are severe, they adversely affect relationships with others.

Epidemiology

Negative emotional behaviors are very common, especially in early childhood. Normally they decrease over time as children learn to control these emotions and to express them verbally rather than behaviorally.

Etiology

Because of their origin, these behaviors are clearly related to the severity of the underlying negative emotions. Therefore, children who are depressed or who are experiencing chronic abuse (see p 45) are more likely to display these behaviors. The severity of these behaviors probably relates to the temperamental trait of negative mood, which may have a significant genetic component (see Children's Responses to Environmental Situations and Potentially Stressful Events preamble, p 31).

DEVELOPMENTAL VARIATION	COMMON DEVELOPMENTAL PRESENTATIONS
V65.49 Negative Emotional Behavior Variation Infants and preschool children typically display negative emotional behaviors when frustrated or irritable. The severity of the behaviors varies depending on temperament (see Children's Responses to Environmental Situations and Potentially Stressful Events preamble, p 31). The degree of difficulty produced by these behaviors depends, in part, on the skill and understanding of the caregivers.	**Infancy** The infant typically cries in response to any frustration, such as hunger or fatigue, or cries for no obvious reason, especially in late afternoon, evening, and nighttime hours. **Early Childhood** The child frequently cries and whines, especially when hungry or tired, is easily frustrated, frequently displays anger by hitting and biting, and has temper tantrums when not given his or her way. **Middle Childhood** The child has temper tantrums, although usually reduced in degree and frequency, and pounds his or her fists or screams when frustrated. **Adolescence** The adolescent may hit objects or slam doors when frustrated and will occasionally curse or scream when angered.

SPECIAL INFORMATION

These negative emotional behaviors are associated with temperamental traits, particularly low adaptability, high intensity, and negative mood (see Children's Responses to Environmental Situations and Potentially Stressful Events preamble, p 31). These behaviors decrease drastically with development, especially as language develops. These behaviors are also especially responsive to discipline.

Environmental factors, especially depression in the parent (see Mental Disorder of Parent, p 46), are associated with negative emotional behaviors in the child. However, these behaviors are more transient than those seen in adjustment disorder (see p 312).

These behaviors increase in situations of environmental stress such as child neglect or physical/sexual abuse (see p 45), but again the behaviors are more transient than those seen in adjustment disorder (see p 312).

As children grow older, their negative emotions and behaviors come under their control. However, outbursts of negative emotional behaviors including temper tantrums are common in early adolescence when adolescents experience frustration in the normal developmental process of separating from their nuclear family and also experience a normal increase in emotional reactiveness. However, a decrease in negative emotional behaviors is associated with normal development in middle to late adolescence.

PROBLEM	COMMON DEVELOPMENTAL PRESENTATIONS
V71.02 Negative Emotional Behavior Problem Negative emotional behaviors that increase (rather than decrease) in intensity, despite appropriate caregiver management, and that begin to interfere with child-adult or peer interactions may be a problem. These behaviors also constitute a problem when combined with other behaviors such as hyperactivity/impulsivity (see Hyperactive/ Impulsive Behaviors cluster, p 93), aggression (see Aggressive/ Oppositional Behavior cluster, p 119), and/or depression (see Sadness and Related Symptoms cluster, p 153). However, the severity and frequency of these behaviors do not meet the criteria for disorder.	**Infancy** The infant flails, pushes away, shakes head, gestures refusal, and dawdles. These actions should not be considered aggressive intentions, but the only way the infant can show frustration or a need for control in response to stress — e.g., separation from parents, intrusive interactions (physical or sexual), overstimulation, loss of a family member, or change in caregivers. **Early Childhood** The child repeatedly, despite appropriate limit setting and proper discipline, has intermittent temper tantrums. These behaviors result in caregiver frustration and can affect interactions with peers. **Middle Childhood** The child has frequent and/or intense responses to frustrations, such as losing in games or not getting his or her way. Negative behaviors begin to affect interaction with peers. **Adolescence** The adolescent has frequent and/or intense reactions to being denied requests and may respond inappropriately to the normal teasing behavior of others. The adolescent is easily frustrated, and the behaviors associated with the frustration interfere with friendships or the completion of age-appropriate tasks.
	SPECIAL INFORMATION
	Intense crying frustrates caregivers. The typical response of caregivers must be assessed in order to evaluate the degree of the problem. The presence of skill deficits as a source of frustration must be considered (e.g., the clumsy child who does not succeed in games in early childhood or in sports in later childhood and adolescence, or the child with a learning disability [see Academic Skills cluster, p 69]).

DISORDER	COMMON DEVELOPMENTAL PRESENTATIONS
Currently there is no specific disorder that is definitely associated with negative emotional behaviors. The symptoms can be components of: **296. Major Depressive Disorder (see Sadness cluster, p 153)** **300.4 Dysthymic Disorder (see Sadness cluster, p 153)** **309.0 Adjustment Disorder With Depressed Mood (see *DSM-IV* Criteria Appendix, p 312)**	
	SPECIAL INFORMATION
	These symptoms can be produced by physical or sexual abuse, serious parental or family conflict, and loss. These environmental issues should always be assessed. Low self-esteem, which is an important part of these disorders, can be the result of frustration and failure associated with learning disorders, mental retardation, communication disorders, and disruptive behavior disorders. These conditions should always be assessed. The diagnosis of adjustment disorder with depressed mood should not be made if the child meets the criteria for major depressive disorder.

DIFFERENTIAL DIAGNOSIS	SPECIAL INFORMATION
General Medical Conditions Any illness (particularly acute illness) that results in anger, loss of self-esteem, or demoralization can lead to negative emotional behaviors. Examples include: Severe physical injury Influenza resulting in prolonged fatigue Acute surgical condition, e.g., appendicitis Prolonged surgical or medical illness In addition, some acute disorders affecting central nervous system (CNS) functioning produces irritability and negative emotional behaviors. Examples include: Encephalitis, viral or bacterial Systemic lupus erythematosus Tumor or injury affecting the limbic system Seizure disorders Degenerative disorders	The negative emotional behaviors should follow, or coincide with, the general medical conditions. Recovery from the illness should result in amelioration of the behavior and the intensity of the symptoms, and impairment should not be sufficient to meet the criteria for an adjustment disorder. Code only the general medical condition if the condition causes the symptoms. Code both if the symptoms are a reaction to the general medical condition. The negative emotional behaviors should follow, or coincide with, the CNS disorder, and recovery from the disorder should result in decrease in the behavior. Code only the CNS condition if the condition causes the symptoms. Code both if the symptoms are a reaction to the general medical condition.
Substances Negative emotional behaviors may be produced particularly by substances that have a depressive effect. Examples include: Alcohol Opioids These behaviors may be produced by stimulant or euphoria-producing substances when the substances are being withdrawn.	The negative emotional behaviors should be seen primarily in association with the substance use and should not remain, or be greatly reduced, when the substance use is terminated. Code only the substance use (see p 135).
Mental Disorders When negative emotional behavior is accompanied by inattention and hyperactive/impulsive behaviors, consider attention-deficit/hyperactivity disorder, hyperactive-impulsive type or combined type (see Hyperactive/Impulsive cluster [p 93], and Inattentive Behaviors cluster [p 103]). When negative emotional behavior is accompanied by oppositional, defiant, and negativistic behaviors, consider oppositional defiant disorder (see Aggressive/Oppositional Behaviors cluster, p 119).	The depressive disorder can be present with other disorders (e.g., major depressive disorder and conduct disorder).

COMMONLY COMORBID CONDITIONS	SPECIAL INFORMATION
Other Comorbid Mental Health Conditions Any of the disruptive behavior disorders commonly coexist with negative emotional behaviors. Examples include: **314.xx** Attention-deficit/hyperactivity disorder **314.01** Combined type **314.01** Predominantly hyperactive/impulsive type **313.81** Oppositional defiant disorder **312.81** Conduct disorder childhood onset **312.82** Conduct disorder adolescent onset	Code the disruptive behavior disorder and negative emotional behavior problem.
Any of the developmental disorders may coexist with negative emotional behaviors. Examples include: **V62.89** Cognitive/adaptive skills problem **317,** Mental retardation **318.x,** **319** **V40.3** Learning problem **315.00** Reading disorder **315.1** Mathematics disorder **315.2** Disorder of written expression **781.3** Developmental coordination problem **315.4** Developmental coordination disorder **V40.1** Speech and language problem **315.31** Expressive language disorder **315.32** Mixed receptive-expressive disorder	Code the developmental problem or disorder and the negative emotional behavior problem. The negative emotional behaviors may be secondary to the low self-esteem produced by these developmental problems. However, the causal association is difficult to establish. Therefore, both conditions should be coded.
Other General Medical Conditions Any static disorder affecting the central nervous system may be associated with negative emotional behaviors. Examples include: Fetal alcohol syndrome Postanoxic brain damage Postencephalitic states Neurocutaneous disorders Post-brain injury states Organic mood disorder	Code both the central nervous system disorder and negative emotional behavior problem when the causality cannot be determined.

Presenting Complaints

not minding

willful ignoring

doing the opposite

arguing

negative attitude

yelling

swearing

mouthing off

fighting

hitting

bullying

Definitions and Symptoms

Opposition indicates the willful refusal to comply with a request from another person, manifest through noncompliant action, argumentative verbalizations, or negative attitudes. Oppositional behavior may also include negativistic verbal or motor behavior that occurs during compliance with requests (e.g., a "bad attitude"). Aggression indicates words or actions that seem intended to harm another person(s) or oneself. Aggression may be instrumental (e.g., using force to obtain a goal); may be frankly hostile (e.g., inflicting pain or destroying property as the primary motive); and/or may be initiated by the child spontaneously (e.g., bullying or retaliatory behavior). Most aggression is directed toward other people or their property, but some may be self-directed. Oppositional behavior peaks during early childhood (at ages 2 or 3 years) and during early adolescence; boys typically exhibit more oppositional behavior than girls. Aggressive behaviors are common in younger children and normally decline with development. Aggressive/oppositional behaviors and particularly defiant and conduct disorders can occur simultaneously with attention-deficit/hyperactivity disorder (ADHD) (see Hyperactive/Impulsive Behaviors cluster, p 93), adjustment disorder, depressive disorder, and bipolar disorders (see Sadness and Related Symptoms cluster, p 153), pervasive developmental disorders (see Social Interaction Behaviors cluster, p 277), posttraumatic stress disorder (PTSD) [see Anxious Symptoms cluster, p 145]), and organic brain disorders. Some of the behaviors can also be seen with pervasive developmental disorder (see Social Interaction Cluster, p 277).

Epidemiology

Aggressive behavior in many cases may show a familial pattern, although this may include both genetic and environmental components. When marked aggression is present, it is important to obtain a family history to identify any history of abuse (see physical and sexual abuse, p 45). The prevalence of conduct disorder ranges from 6% to 16% for males and 2% to 9% for females under 18 years of age. Rates of oppositional defiant disorder for males under age 18 years range from 2% to 16%. The rates of both conduct disorder and oppositional defiant disorder vary widely depending on the nature of the population sampled and the methods of ascertainment used.

Etiology

The following factors may predispose the individual to the development of conduct disorder and oppositional defiant disorder: parental rejection and neglect, difficult infant temperament, inconsistent child-rearing practices with harsh discipline, physical or sexual abuse, lack of supervision, early institutional living, frequent changes of caregivers, association with a delinquent peer group, and certain kinds of familial psychopathology such as parental criminality or antisocial personality disorder.

DEVELOPMENTAL VARIATION	COMMON DEVELOPMENTAL PRESENTATIONS
V65.49 Aggressive/Oppositional Variation **Oppositionality** Mild opposition with mild negative impact is a normal developmental variation. Mild opposition may occur several times a day for a short period. Mild negative impact occurs when no one is hurt, no property is damaged, and parents do not significantly alter their plans.	**Infancy** The infant sometimes flails, pushes away, shakes head, gestures refusal, and dawdles. These behaviors may not be considered aggressive intentions, but the only way the infant can show frustration or a need for control in response to stress, e.g., separation from parents, intrusive interactions (physical or sexual), overstimulation, loss of family member, change in caregivers. **Early Childhood** The child's negative behavior includes saying "no" as well as all of the above behaviors but with increased sophistication and purposefulness. The child engages in brief arguments, uses bad language, purposely does the opposite of what is asked, and procrastinates. **Middle Childhood** The child's oppositional behaviors include all of the above behaviors, elaborately defying doing chores, making up excuses, using bad language, displaying negative attitudes, and using gestures that indicate refusal. **Adolescence** The adolescent's oppositional behaviors include engaging in more abstract verbal arguments, demanding reasons for requests, and often giving excuses.
	SPECIAL INFORMATION
	Oppositional behavior occurs in common situations such as getting dressed, picking up toys, during meals, or at bedtime. In early childhood, these situations broaden to include preschool and home life. In middle childhood, an increase in school-related situations occurs. In adolescence, independence-related issues become important.

DEVELOPMENTAL VARIATION	COMMON DEVELOPMENTAL PRESENTATIONS
V65.4 Aggressive/Oppositional Variation **Aggression** In order to assert a growing sense of self, nearly all children display some amount of aggression, particularly during periods of rapid developmental transition. Aggression tends to decline normatively with development. Aggression is more common in younger children, who lack self-regulatory skills, than in older children, who internalize familial and societal standards and learn to use verbal mediation to delay gratification. Children may shift normatively to verbal opposition with development. Mild aggression may occur several times per week, with minimal negative impact.	**Infancy** The infant's aggressive behaviors include crying, refusing to be nurtured, kicking, and biting, but are usually not persistent. **Early Childhood** The child's aggressive behaviors include some grabbing toys, hitting siblings and others, kicking, and being verbally abusive to others, but usually responds to parental reprimand. **Middle Childhood** The child's aggressive behaviors include some engaging in all of the above behaviors, with more purposefulness, "getting even" for perceived injustice, inflicting pain on others, using profane language, and bullying and hitting peers. The behaviors are intermittent and there is usually provocation. **Adolescence** The adolescent exhibits overt physical aggression less frequently, curses, mouths off, and argues, usually with provocation.
	SPECIAL INFORMATION
	In middle childhood, more aggression and self-defense occur at school and with peers. During adolescence, aggressive and oppositional behaviors blend together in many cases.

PROBLEM	COMMON DEVELOPMENTAL PRESENTATIONS
V71.02 Aggressive/Oppositional Problem **Oppositionality** The child will display some of the symptoms listed for oppositional defiant disorder (see p 123). The frequency of the opposition occurs enough to be bothersome to parents or supervising adults, but not often enough to be considered a disorder.	**Infancy** The infant screams a lot, runs away from parents a lot, and ignores requests. **Early Childhood** The child ignores requests frequently enough to be a problem, dawdles frequently enough to be a problem, argues back while doing chores, throws tantrums when asked to do some things, messes up the house on purpose, has a negative attitude many days, and runs away from parents on several occasions. **Middle Childhood** The child intermittently tries to annoy others such as turning up the radio on purpose, making up excuses, begins to ask for reasons why when given commands, and argues for longer times. These behaviors occur frequently enough to be bothersome to the family. **Adolescence** The adolescent argues back often, frequently has a negative attitude, sometimes makes obscene gestures, and argues and procrastinates in more intense and sophisticated ways.
	SPECIAL INFORMATION
	All children occasionally defy adult requests for compliance, particularly the requests of their parents. More opposition is directed toward mothers than fathers. Boys display opposition more often than girls and their opposition tends to be expressed by behaviors that are more motor oriented. The most intense opposition occurs at the apex of puberty for boys and the onset of menarche for girls.

PROBLEM	COMMON DEVELOPMENTAL PRESENTATIONS
V71.02 Aggressive/Oppositional Problem **Aggression** When levels of aggression and hostility interfere with family routines, begin to engender negative responses from peers or teachers, and/or cause disruption at school, problematic status is evident. The negative impact is moderate. People change routines; property begins to be more seriously damaged. The child will display some of the symptoms listed for conduct disorder (see p 124) but not enough to warrant the diagnosis of the disorder. However, the behaviors are not sufficiently intense to qualify for a behavioral disorder.	**Infancy** The infant bites, kicks, cries, and pulls hair fairly frequently. **Early Childhood** The child frequently grabs others' toys, shouts, hits or punches siblings and others, and is verbally abusive. **Middle Childhood** The child gets into fights intermittently in school or in the neighborhood, swears or uses bad language sometimes in inappropriate settings, hits or otherwise hurts self when angry or frustrated. **Adolescence** The adolescent intermittently hits others, uses bad language, is verbally abusive, may display some inappropriate suggestive sexual behaviors.
	SPECIAL INFORMATION
	Problem levels of aggressive behavior may run in families. When marked aggression is present, the assessor must examine the family system, the types of behaviors modeled, and the possibility of abusive interactions.

DISORDER	COMMON DEVELOPMENTAL PRESENTATIONS
313.81 Oppositional Defiant Disorder Hostile, defiant behavior towards others of at least 6 months' duration that is developmentally inappropriate. • often loses temper • often argues with adults • often actively defies or refuses to comply with adults' requests or rules • often deliberately annoys people • often blames others for his or her mistakes or misbehavior • is often touchy or easily annoyed by others • is often angry and resentful • is often spiteful or vindictive (see *DSM-IV* Criteria Appendix, p 335)	**Infancy** It is not possible to make the diagnosis. **Early Childhood** The child is extremely defiant, refuses to do as asked, mouths off, throws tantrums. **Middle Childhood** The child is very rebellious, refusing to comply with reasonable requests, argues often, and annoys other people on purpose. **Adolescence** The adolescent is frequently rebellious, has severe arguments, follows parents around while arguing, is defiant, has negative attitudes, is unwilling to compromise, and may precociously use alcohol, tobacco, or illicit drugs.

DISORDER	COMMON DEVELOPMENTAL PRESENTATIONS
312.81 Conduct Disorder Childhood Onset **312.82 Conduct Disorder Adolescent Onset** A repetitive and persistent pattern of behavior in which the basic rights of others or major age-appropriate societal norms or rules are violated. Onset may occur as early as age 5 to 6 years, but is usually in late childhood or early adolescence. The behaviors harm others and break societal rules including stealing, fighting, destroying property, lying, truancy, and running away from home. (see *DSM-IV* Criteria Appendix, p 322) **309.3 Adjustment Disorder With Disturbance of Conduct** (see *DSM-IV* Criteria Appendix, p 312) **312.9 Disruptive Behavior Disorder, NOS** (see *DSM-IV* Criteria Appendix, p 325)	**Infancy** It is not possible to make the diagnosis. **Early Childhood** Symptoms are rarely of such a quality or intensity to be able to diagnose the disorder. **Middle Childhood** The child often may exhibit some of the following behaviors: lies, steals, fights with peers with and without weapons, is cruel to people or animals, may display some inappropriate sexual activity, bullies, engages in destructive acts, violates rules, acts deceitful, is truant from school, and has academic difficulties. **Adolescence** The adolescent displays delinquent, aggressive behavior, harms people and property more often than in middle childhood, exhibits deviant sexual behavior, uses illegal drugs, is suspended/expelled from school, has difficulties with the law, acts reckless, runs away from home, is destructive, violates rules, has problems adjusting at work, and has academic difficulties.
	SPECIAL INFORMATION
	The best predictor of aggression that will reach the level of a disorder is a diversity of antisocial behaviors exhibited at an early age; clinicians should be alert to this factor. Oppositional defiant disorder usually becomes evident before age 8 years and usually not later than early adolescence. Oppositional defiant disorder is more prevalent in males than in females before puberty, but rates are probably equal after puberty. The occurrence of the following negative environmental factors may increase the likelihood, severity, and negative prognosis of conduct disorder: parental rejection and neglect (see p 46), inconsistent management with harsh discipline, physical or sexual child abuse (see p 45), lack of supervision, early institutional living (see p 45), frequent changes of caregivers (see p 48), and association with delinquent peer group. Suicidal ideation, suicide attempts, and completed suicide occur at a higher than expected rate (see Suicidal Thoughts or Behaviors cluster, p 165). If the criteria are met for both oppositional defiant disorder and conduct disorder, only code conduct disorder.

DIFFERENTIAL DIAGNOSIS	SPECIAL INFORMATION
	While developmental disorders such as fetal alcohol syndrome are likely to be the cause of some underlying aggressive symptoms, the underlying conditions are rarely correctable so it is difficult to establish the general medical condition diagnoses as the cause. Therefore it is better to utilize the co-diagnoses outline in the section below.
Substances Any substance that produces depression or heightened excitement may result in an increase in aggressive/oppositional behaviors. Examples include: Alcohol Opiates Cocaine Stimulants PCPs Steroids	The aggressive/oppositional behaviors should subside with termination of the substance use. The reverse situation frequently occurs in that children with conduct and oppositional disorder are at higher risk of substance abuse. These conditions may cause problems but it is not likely that they cause symptoms at a disorder level. Substance withdrawal can cause depressive effects (see Negative Emotional Mood and Sadness and Related Symptoms cluster [see pp 113 and 153] as well as Anxious Symptoms cluster [see p 145]).
Mental Disorders Mental disorders associated with depressive symptoms may produce aggressive behaviors associated with irritable mood. If the mental disorder occurs following or simultaneously with the aggressive behavior and treatment of the mood disorder corrects the aggressive/oppositional behaviors, diagnose only the mental disorder. Examples include: **296.xx** Major depressive disorder **296.5x** Bipolar I disorder, most recent episode depressed **300.4** Dysthymic disorder	More than one disorder can occur simultaneously and should be coded if one disorder is not causing the symptoms suggesting the disorder.

COMMONLY COMORBID CONDITIONS	SPECIAL INFORMATION
Other Comorbid Mental Health Conditions Mental disorders associated with depression can coexist with an aggressive/oppositional behavior problem or disorder. Examples include: **296.xx** Major depressive disorder **296.5x** Bipolar I disorder, most recent episode depressed **300.4** Dysthymic disorder	The mental health disorder should have been present before, or at the same time, as the aggressive/oppositional behaviors. Code both conditions.
Other General Medical Conditions Any acute illness, especially requiring hospitalization Any severe injury Sickle cell disease, especially during crises Cystic fibrosis Diabetes mellitus	Any acute or chronic medical condition that results in lowered self-esteem, demoralization, or developmental regression may result in increased aggressive/oppositional behaviors as a reaction to the condition. Code only the general medical condition if it is the cause of these symptoms. If, as is most commonly the case, the symptoms are a reaction to the medical situation, code either the disorder or adjustment disorder with disturbance of conduct. Since the behaviors are likely to be a reaction to the medical condition, it is appropriate to code both conditions.

Presenting Complaints

lying
cheating
stealing
destroying property
truancy
fire-setting
substance abuse

Definition and Symptoms

Secretive or covert antisocial behaviors are those actions that violate the rights of others or oppose society's ethical or legal standards, and occur surreptitiously or in the absence of adult supervision. Although these behaviors often occur together with overt physical and verbal aggression in children at risk for delinquent behavior, the covert behaviors appear as a separate dimension in studies of antisocial acts. Secretive antisocial behaviors are significant because they typically violate the rights or property of others. The commission of individual antisocial actions does not automatically assume problematic or disordered functioning. However, when persistent patterns of secretive antisocial behaviors occur, there is often an accompanying pattern of familial and psychological indicators that signify the need for intervention.

A crucial issue with regard to the secretive antisocial behaviors is their detection. In general, detection becomes more difficult as the child develops and becomes more sophisticated in the planning of surreptitious actions. In many cases, however, covert behaviors are performed impulsively, without much forethought, which may make detection easier. It is important to note that the performance of covert antisocial behaviors in a child with significant levels of inattentive, impulsive, and hyperactive behaviors (attention-deficit/hyperactivity disorder [see Hyperactive/Impulsive Behaviors cluster, p 93, and Inattentive Behaviors cluster, p 103]) is particularly predictive of later delinquency. Children themselves are a crucial source of information about the commission of these behaviors because the clandestine nature of most of these actions makes it difficult for adults to be accurate appraisers. Similar to overt antisocial actions, the magnitude or intensity of the secretive behaviors, the frequency of their display, and their cross-situational nature are of critical prognostic importance. Several longitudinal investigations have documented that it is the presence of a variety of antisocial behaviors performed at an early age that best predicts subsequent delinquency and antisocial personality in later life.

A common developmental sequence for those youngsters headed toward more serious antisocial behavior and aggression is one in which a pattern of hostile, irritable, and defiant behavior emerges in early childhood (typically diagnosable as oppositional defiant disorder). By the transition to middle childhood, fighting and petty stealing typically appear, presaging the more serious antisocial behaviors associated with conduct disorder (severe property destruction, assault, forced sexual activity).

Although for many youngsters substance abuse is associated with the development of both overt and covert antisocial behaviors, for another subgroup there appears to be a developmental pathway that leads to substance use in the absence of other indicators of antisocial behavior.

Epidemiology

Sound epidemiologic data on secretive antisocial behaviors are sparse, mainly because of low base rates and the clandestine nature of these acts. Data from adult informants and from child self-report measures do reveal, however, that unlike overt aggressive behaviors, which typically decrease throughout childhood, secretive actions show a gradual increase through childhood and early adolescence. Furthermore, some degree of, for example, cheating in school, lying to parents about misbehavior, or destroying materials during a tantrum may be considered normative. Concern is indicated when a pattern of more severe or more frequent antisocial behaviors begins to develop. At a disorder level the secretive antisocial behaviors are found as a part of the symptoms of conduct disorder. The prevalence of conduct disorder for males under age 18 years ranges from 6% to 16%; for females, rates range from 2% to 9%. Because some signs of secretive antisocial behaviors tend to emerge early in the developmental sequence, the early tracking of these behaviors is essential.

DEVELOPMENTAL VARIATION	COMMON DEVELOPMENTAL PRESENTATIONS
V65.49 Secretive Antisocial Behaviors Variation As noted in the preliminary comments, secretive antisocial behaviors appear at low base rates during early and middle childhood, with a normative increase toward adolescence. Mild levels of cheating, lying, and taking of small objects are usually not of clinical concern during childhood, and some evidence exists that some experimentation with alcohol and substances in adolescence does not portend maladjustment.	**Infancy** Not relevant at this age. **Early Childhood** The child occasionally cheats during games, lies to deny responsibility for misbehavior, and secretly takes small amounts of money from parents. **Middle Childhood** The child occasionally rips and tears papers during a tantrum, cheats on tests at school, and has a single episode of minor shoplifting. **Adolescence** The adolescent occasionally experiments with drinking alcohol or smoking marijuana.
	SPECIAL INFORMATION
	The occasional occurrence of and the lack of harm resulting from selected covert actions signal normative, as opposed to problematic, levels of covert behavior.

PROBLEM	COMMON DEVELOPMENTAL PRESENTATIONS
V71.02 Secretive Antisocial Behaviors Problem Secretive antisocial behaviors become problematic when their rates, intensity, and consequences increase and when parents or caregivers begin to suspect a pattern of lying to hide the offending actions.	**Infancy** Not relevant at this age. **Early Childhood** The child lies intentionally to escape punishment, becomes fascinated with matches, and rips up papers after arguments. **Middle Childhood** The child sometimes shoplifts relatively unsubstantial items and hides parents' belongings following stressful incident. May occasionally take money from parents or others. **Adolescence** The adolescent sometimes will shoplift relatively unsubstantial items, uses keys to scratch paint off cars, regularly creates graffiti on walls, sometimes causes mild damage to property, and begins to use alcohol on a repetitive basis but not to a sufficient degree to warrant a conduct disorder or substance abuse disorder diagnosis.
	SPECIAL INFORMATION
	For a problem, as opposed to a disorder, behaviors are still not frequent and levels of harm are relatively low. These behaviors can be associated with dysfunctional family interactions and/or patterns of abuse (see physical or sexual abuse, p 45). These possibilities should always be evaluated.

DISORDER	COMMON DEVELOPMENTAL PRESENTATIONS
312.81 Conduct Disorder Childhood Onset **312.82 Conduct Disorder Adolescent Onset** When levels of secretive antisocial behavior are persistent and typically associated with overt aggression as well, conduct disorder should be diagnosed. The criteria for conduct disorder includes both overt aggression and secretive anti-social behaviors. The diagnosis requires at least three of the conduct disorders symptoms causing a sufficient degree of impairment. This usually entails a per-sistent pattern of antisocial activity that debases the basic rights of others or major age-appropriate societal norms or rules are violated. (see *DSM-IV* Criteria Appendix, p 322) **309.3 Adjustment Disorder With Disturbance of Conduct** (see *DSM-IV* Criteria Appendix, p 312) **312.9 Disruptive Behavior Disorder, NOS** (see *DSM-IV* Criteria Appendix, p 325)	**Infancy** Not relevant at this age. **Early Childhood** The child persistently demonstrates some of the following behaviors: lies, steals, plays with matches, starts fires, and destroys property. **Middle Childhood** The child persistently demonstrates some of the following behaviors: lies, cheats constantly at school, steals chronically, persistently plays with matches, intentionally starts fires with the intention of causing serious damage, is truant, experiments with alcohol and other substances, and willfully destroys property at home, at school, or in the neighborhood. **Adolescence** The adolescent has the same behaviors as in middle childhood, only with greater frequency and/or intensity.

SPECIAL INFORMATION

A pattern of diverse antisocial behaviors occurring at an early age predicts delinquency, comorbid ADHD, and persistent antisocial behavior and it is more typically found in males.

Distant and/or discordant family interactions (see Other family rela-tionship problems, p 45), poor parental monitoring of the youth's behavior, neglectful and physically or sexually abusive interactions (see p 45), lack of supervision, early institutional living (see p 45), frequent changes of caregivers (see p 48), and association with delinquent peer group are associated with development of persis-tent patterns of secretive antisocial behaviors and conduct disorder.

The risk for legal involvement is clearly associated with antisocial behavior, rising in direct proportion to the severity and intensity of the behavior. Suicide ideation, suicide attempts, and completed suicide occur at a higher than expected rate (see Suicidal Thoughts or Behaviors cluster, p 165).

The secretive antisocial behaviors frequently occur simultaneously and cannot be separated from aggressive behaviors (see Aggres-sive/Oppositional Behaviors cluster, p 119).

DIFFERENTIAL DIAGNOSIS	SPECIAL INFORMATION
General Medical Conditions	Reactions to general medical conditions, particularly when they lower self-esteem, can cause an increase in secretive antisocial behavior, but there are no specific causal conditions.
Substances Examples include: Marijuana Alcohol Cocaine Phencyclidine Heroin and other narcotics	In some cases, a chronic pattern of secretive behaviors may occur simultaneously with the substance use; in others, stealing and/or assault may follow the establishment of substance dependence. In adolescents with a pattern of substance dependence, a lifestyle marked by repetitive stealing (with or without confrontation of the victim) may ensue, with the goal of obtaining money for purchase of additional substances. Code only the substance use/abuse.
Mental Disorders 300.3 Obsessive-compulsive disorder 296.xx Major depressive disorder 309.3 Adjustment disorder, with disturbance of conduct 300.4 Dysthymic disorder 307.51 Bulimia nervosa	Occasionally, severe obsessive-compulsive disorder may lead to compulsive stealing. Mood disorders (depression, bipolar disorder) may be associated with antisocial behaviors. Currently little is known about the causal links between mood disorders and the display of conduct disorder (including persistent secretive antisocial behaviors). In some youngsters, the mood disorder appears primary. Code only the mental disorder.

COMMONLY COMORBID CONDITIONS	SPECIAL INFORMATION
Other Comorbid Mental Health Conditions Disruptive behavior disorders, developmental disorders, and depressive disorders may coexist with secretive antisocial behaviors. Examples include: 314.xx Attention-deficit/hyperactivity disorder (ADHD) 314.01 Predominantly hyperactive-impulsive type 314.01 Combined type 313.81 Oppositional defiant disorder 315.xx Learning disorders 315.xx, Communication disorder 307.xx 300.02 Generalized anxiety disorder 296.xx Major depressive disorder 305 Substance abuse disorder 300.4 Dysthymic disorder 307.51 Bulimia nervosa 300.3 Obsessive-compulsive disorder	The impulsivity and poor judgment of ADHD, when linked with antisocial behavior, presages a particularly poor prognosis. Code both (or more) disorders. ADHD, particularly the predominantly hyperactive-impulsive and combined subtypes, is frequently linked with the subsequent development of secretive (as well as overtly aggressive) antisocial behavior patterns.

SUBSTANCE USE/ABUSE

SUBSTANCE USE/ABUSE

SUBSTANCE USE/ABUSE

Presenting Complaints

drinks alcohol

smokes marijuana

sniffs glue

takes illegal drugs

smokes cigarettes

inappropriately uses medications

Definitions and Symptoms

These behaviors involve the taking of any substance, such as alcohol or other drugs, that are either prohibited for children or illegal at any age. These behaviors also include taking medications that have not been prescribed, such as the unauthorized use of steroids by athletes. Substance use/abuse is not usually an issue until at least ages 10 to 11 years, and becomes an increasingly prevalent problem as adolescence progresses. Excessive use of alcohol is always a problem; any use of this substance is a significant problem in some cultures and communities. The unauthorized use of prescription drugs is always a problem. Underage cigarette smoking is always a *medical* health concern, but in *some* adolescents, it may be a marker for the beginning of a pattern of more serious substance use or misuse. Cigarette use can lead to nicotine dependence, resulting in an increased need for cigarettes (chain smoking) and restricting activities based on the need to avoid access when smoking is restricted.

Substance use/abuse by children is clearly associated with a number of environmental factors such as poverty (see p 51), the experience of physical or sexual abuse (see p 45), and the negative influence of peers or family members. Substance abuse is also associated with behavior disorders (e.g., mood, anxiety, learning) and those disorders that result in poor self-esteem such as conduct disorder or attention-deficit/hyperactivity disorder.

Cultural, religious, and family values and practices must be considered in evaluating the severity of substance use problems. In an environment that strongly prohibits any use of substances, even occasional use of a substance may indicate a significant problem. However, in a community or family where, for example, alcohol use is acceptable, occasional experimentation may be within the normal experience, but repeated or excessive use even in those environments is a problem.

Etiology

Substances are usually used because they have an effect that is considered pleasurable, although the effects often last for only brief periods, and/or because they reduce or distract from painful feelings or thoughts. Peer pressure is also an important reason children use substances. Studies have repeatedly demonstrated that a pattern of substance abuse problems typically begins with occasional use of one or two substances with a gradual increase in the number of different substances used and the amount consumed. Children of substance-abusing parents are at an increased risk to develop substance-related problems.

DEVELOPMENTAL VARIATION	COMMON DEVELOPMENTAL PRESENTATIONS

V65.49 Substance Use Variation

The occasional use of illegal substances in the context of experimentation (i.e., in the presence of a peer group all engaging in the same behavior) may be a part of late school age or adolescent behavior. What constitutes nonproblematic experimentation should be judged in the context of the community's norms, legal statutes, and the social/cultural milieu. For example, experimentation might be common in large city environments, but highly unlikely in a more rural, close-knit, or religious community. The degree to which this behavior poses a problem is also related to the sensitivity of the caregiver to this kind of behavior. Some parents may see a single episode of substance use as a major concern, while others may not react to several episodes.

Infancy and Early Childhood
Not relevant at this age.

Middle Childhood
The child may occasionally try a substance when dared by peers, but this should initially be treated as a problem unless it proves to be an isolated incident.

Adolescence
The adolescent may try a substance such as marijuana or alcohol at a party on a one-time basis with friends "just to see what it is like."

SPECIAL INFORMATION

This issue is not usually relevant in infancy or early childhood, except in situations of passive exposure secondary to use by a caregiver, such as an infant being exposed to crack cocaine because of adult use. There have also been occasional reports of a parent giving unprescribed alcohol to an infant in order to quiet the child. This should be considered a possible incidence of child abuse or neglect (see Neglect, p 46). Also, toddlers sometimes mistakenly drink alcohol kept in the house, in which case it is considered a poison. Experimentation with substances is more likely in some cultures and environmental situations, and the appropriateness of its use must be judged accordingly. Children are more frequently exposed to substance use in urban environments. In some communities, the occasional use of alcohol or the smoking of cigarettes and/or marijuana may be an expression of late school age or adolescent development.

If the substance use is associated with a social/emotional problem in the child, or if it occurs while the child is alone, it is less likely to represent experimentation. It is also of greater concern if the peer group that exerts the pressure to use substances is a behaviorally disturbed group. Those children and adolescents who are impulsive (see Hyperactive/Impulsive Behaviors cluster, p 93) are more likely to experiment. Onset of use before age 15 years has the greatest risk for long-lasting dysfunctional patterns of abuse. Increased susceptibility to alcoholism is seen in sons of alcoholic fathers and the male twin of an alcoholic sibling. A family history or a cultural history of substance abuse increases the level of concern. Low self-esteem, low self-confidence, and lack of assertiveness are important risk factors, increasing the likelihood of concern.

Adolescents may try alcohol, cigarettes, or marijuana (rarely other illegal drugs) in situations of group/peer pressure such as at parties or other gatherings. In some cultures, alcohol and, less frequently, certain other drugs, are freely offered to the adolescent in the home. Regular use of these substances, however, except for culturally sanctioned use, is not within the range of expected behavior.

PROBLEM	COMMON DEVELOPMENTAL PRESENTATIONS
V71.09 Substance Use Problem When an illegal substance is used more than once but has not become a repeated behavior and has not significantly impaired function even occasionally, it is a problem. Also, if substance use occurs while the child is alone or in the context of behavioral/emotional difficulties, it is also a problem. Use of illegal drugs is a problem. Any unauthorized use of prescription drugs is a problem.	**Infancy and Early Childhood** Not relevant at this age. **Middle Childhood** The child may engage in more than one-time use of substances during peer group activity and may occasionally use alcohol or marijuana more than one time. The occasional occurrence of dysfunctional behavior (e.g., memory loss) indicates a problem. **Adolescence** The adolescent uses alcohol or marijuana on more than a one-time basis (i.e., once a month or more), occasionally uses substances alone or because of behavioral/emotional problems, occasionally experiences impaired memory or motor functions as a result of substance use, uses drugs on one or a few occasions.

	SPECIAL INFORMATION
	A problem of substance use that is associated with a stressful period in the adolescent's life may go away when the stressful period is over. Any child younger than 11 who even experiments with drugs should be evaluated for a disorder. A significant change in the child/adolescent's social milieu may have an important favorable impact on the substance use problem. For example, the adolescent who becomes involved in a religious group may discontinue substance use.

DISORDER	COMMON DEVELOPMENTAL PRESENTATIONS
305.xx Substance Abuse Disorder **303.xx, 304.xx Substance Dependence** A disorder should be considered when the child experiences tolerance, withdrawal, and the substance is taken often in large amounts and over a longer period of time than intended. The substance use takes up a significant portion of his or her activities, interfering with other activities, and is difficult to stop. **305.xx Substance Abuse** Recurrent substance abuse resulting in failure to fulfill major role obligations at home or school and use in physical hazardous situations, resulting in legal problems, despite causing persistent and recurrent social and interpersonal problems. **305.xx Substance Intoxication** The development of a reversible substance-specific syndrome due to recent ingestion of (or exposure to) a substance, resulting in clinically significant maladaptive behavioral and psychological changes. **292.0 Substance Withdrawal** The development of a substance-specific syndrome due to the cessation of (or reduction in) substance use that has been heavy and prolonged, causing clinically significant distress and impairment in important areas of function.	**Infancy and Early Childhood** Not relevant at this age. **Middle Childhood** The child has a repeated pattern of alcohol or other drug use, experiences impaired functioning from substance use, has a decrease in grades at school. **Adolescence** The adolescent repeatedly uses alcohol and/or marijuana or other drugs and use is associated with impaired functioning at school, at home, or with peers. **SPECIAL INFORMATION** A substance abuse disorder associated with an ongoing emotional problem may go away when the emotional problem is treated. The possibility of associated mental disorders is high. It is important to assess the child for dual or multiple diagnoses. The coding system for substance-related disorders is complex and is linked to specific substances. In order to code the specific substance, please refer to the *DSM-IV* Criteria Appendix (p 349) for specific codes to use.

DIFFERENTIAL DIAGNOSIS	SPECIAL INFORMATION
General Medical Conditions — Examples include: Any medical condition that results in the acute impairment of memory or motor function can be confused with the effects of substance use. Examples include: Diabetic ketoacidosis Hypoglycemia Meningoencephalitis Acute lupus erythematosus Kidney or liver failure Trauma	This confusion of symptom causation is obviously more likely when the medical symptom occurs in a known substance-abusing person or when the medical condition develops in the context where substance use is expected, e.g., at a party or bar. Code only the medical condition.
Substances Not relevant.	
Mental Disorders Mental disorders resulting in acute, confusional states may be confused with substance use/abuse problem or disorder. Examples include: **295.00** Schizophrenia Organic brain syndrome	Code only the mental disorder if there is no evidence (e.g., toxicology tests) of substance use.

COMMONLY COMORBID CONDITIONS	SPECIAL INFORMATION
Other Comorbid Mental Health Conditions Any mental health condition that leads to low self-esteem or demoralization can lead to substance use/abuse. Often the substance use alleviates the emotional problem, at least in the short term. **314.xx** Attention-deficit/hyperactivity disorder **314.01** Predominantly hyperactive-impulsive type **314.01** Combined type **315.00** Reading disorder **315.1** Mathematical disorder **315.2** Disorder of written expression **313.81** Oppositional defiant disorder **312.81** Conduct disorder childhood onset **312.82** Conduct disorder adolescent onset **300.2** Generalized anxiety disorders **309.81** Posttraumatic stress disorder **296.xx** Major depressive disorder **300.4** Dysthymic disorder	Though the substance use/abuse is thought to stem from the mental health condition, both conditions coexist and treatment for both conditions is usually necessary. Code both the substance use/abuse and the mental health condition. Specific substance use codes are listed in *DSM-IV* Criteria Appendix (p 349).
Other General Medical Conditions Any chronic illness that results in poor self-esteem or demoralization may be associated with substance use/abuse. Examples include: Cystic fibrosis Sickle cell disease Scoliosis Chronic disfiguring dermatitis Disfiguring birth defect Chronic asthma Chronic diabetes	Though the medical condition precedes and is thought to lead to substance use/abuse, both conditions are thought to coexist. Code both the medical condition and the substance use/abuse. Specific substance use codes are listed in the *DSM-IV* Criteria Appendix, p 349. Drug use that includes intravenous use places the child at risk for human immunodeficiency virus infection.

Emotions and Moods

Anxious Symptoms

Sadness and Related Symptoms

Ritualistic, Obsessive, Compulsive Symptoms

Suicidal Thoughts or Behaviors

Presenting Complaints

anxiety

tachycardia

shortness of breath

fear

sense of "going crazy"

separation problems

scared

repetitive play

sleep difficulties

shyness

palpitation

dizziness

refuses to attend school

sense of impending death

nervousness and worry

tremulousness

avoidant behavior

hypervigilance

social withdrawal

Definitions and Symptoms

Anxiety is a normal response to sudden, threatening changes facing an individual, which may include real danger or perceived loss of self-esteem or control. Although the specific manifestations of anxiety vary from individual to individual, generally there are signs of motor tension, autonomic hyperactivity, worry about future events, and wariness. When symptoms of anxiety are persistent, causing distress and dysfunction, there is a need for treatment and when accompanied with suicidal feelings, substance abuse, or other self-destructive behaviors, there are serious risk factors indicating the need for immediate treatment. Often anxiety is concurrent with feelings of depression. Rituals or ruminations may also be present in some cases. In evaluating the seriousness of anxiety, observe whether or not the anxiety interferes with normal daily functioning, is inappropriate for the child's age, or is out of proportion for the situation. If anxiety persists despite efforts to control it, or in the presence of usual comforting persons, professional help is indicated. Anxious symptoms may also be the result of a wide variety of medical disorders and psychoactive substances (see differential diagnosis).

Epidemiology

The lifetime prevalence rates for the disorders of anxiety are: generalized anxiety, 5%; social phobia, 3% to 13%; specific phobia, 10% to 11%; separation anxiety, 4%.

Etiology

Anxiety may be triggered as an instinctual (reflex) response to pain from a sudden or noxious event, or it may occur in anticipation of a feared event or in response to a traumatic event. Anxiety may be learned by repeated exposure to unpleasant events or by observing others reacting fearfully. It may be a reaction to an unpleasant or unfamiliar bodily sensation. Anxiety disorders appear with greater than expected frequency in some families and may have a genetic predisposition.

DEVELOPMENTAL VARIATION	COMMON DEVELOPMENTAL PRESENTATIONS
V65.49 Anxious Variation Fears and worries are experienced that are appropriate for developmental age and do not affect normal development. Transient anxious responses to stressful events occur in an otherwise healthy child and they do not affect normal development.	**Infancy** Normal fears of noises, heights, and loss of physical support are present at birth. Fear of separation from parent figures and fear of strangers are normal symptoms during the first years of life. The latter peaks at 8 to 9 months. Feeding or sleeping changes are possible in the first year. Transient developmental regressions occur after the first year. Scary dreams may occur. **Early Childhood** By age 3 years, children can separate temporarily from a parent with minimal crying or clinging behaviors. Children described as shy or slow to warm up to others may be anxious in new situations. Specific fears of thunder, medical settings, and animals are present. **Middle Childhood** In middle childhood, a child with anxious symptoms may present with motor responses (trembling voice, nail biting, thumb sucking) or physiologic responses (headache, recurrent abdominal pain, unexplained limb pain, vomiting, breathlessness). Normally these should be transient and associated with appropriate stressors. Transient fears may occur after frightening events, such as a scary movie. These should be relieved easily with reassurance. **Adolescence** Adolescents may be shy, avoid usual pursuits, fear separation from friends, and be reluctant to engage in new experiences. Risk-taking behaviors, such as experimentation with drugs or impulsive sexual behavior, may be seen.
	SPECIAL INFORMATION
	Clinicians should attempt to identify any potential stressful events that may have precipitated the anxiety symptoms (see Environmental Situations Defined, p 31). Difficulty falling asleep, frequent night awakenings, tantrums and aggressiveness, and excessive napping may reflect anxiety.

PROBLEM	COMMON DEVELOPMENTAL PRESENTATIONS
V40.2 Anxiety Problem An anxiety problem involves excessive worry or fearfulness that causes significant distress in the child. However, the behaviors are not sufficiently intense to qualify for an anxiety disorder or adjustment disorder with anxious mood.	**Infancy and Early Childhood** In infancy and early childhood, anxiety problems usually present with a more prolonged distress at separation or as sleep and feeding difficulties including anxious clinging when not separating. **Middle Childhood** In middle childhood, anxiety may be manifest as sleep problems, fears of animals, natural disasters, and medical care, worries about being the center of attention, sleep-overs, class trips, and the future (see Sadness and Related Symptoms cluster, p 153). Anxiety may involve some somatic symptoms such as tachycardia, shortness of breath, sweating, choking, nausea, dryness, and chest pain (see Pain/Somatic Complaints cluster, p 173). Environmental stress may be associated with regression (loss of developmental skills), social withdrawal, agitation/hyperactivity, or repetitive reenactment of a traumatic event through play. These symptoms should not be severe enough to warrant the diagnoses of a disorder and should resolve with the alleviation of the stressors. **Adolescence** In adolescence, anxiety may be manifest as sleep problems and fears of medical care and animals. Worries about class performance, participation in sports, and acceptance by peers may be present. Environmental stress may be associated with social withdrawal, boredom (see Sadness and Related Symptoms cluster, p 153), aggressiveness, or some risk-taking behavior (e.g., indiscriminate sexual behavior, drug use, or recklessness).
	SPECIAL INFORMATION
	Anxiety problems have a number of different clinical presentations *including* persistent worries about multiple areas in the child's life, excessive or unreasonable fear of a specific object or situation, fear of situations in which the child has to perform or be scrutinized by others, excessive worry about separation from parents, or anxiety following a significant, identifiable stressor. Separation difficulties may be prolonged if inadvertently rewarded by parents and can result in a separation anxiety disorder. Parental response to the child's distress or anxiety is a key factor in the assessment of anxiety problems. The extent of the child's anxiety may be difficult to assess and the primary care clinicians should err on the side of referral to a mental health clinician if there is uncertainty about the severity of the condition.

DISORDER	COMMON DEVELOPMENTAL PRESENTATIONS
300.02 Generalized Anxiety Disorder This disorder is characterized by at least 6 months of persistent and excessive anxiety and worry. Excessive and persistent worry occurs across a multitude of domains or situations, such as school work, sports, or social performance, and is associated with impaired functioning. The disorder is often associated with somatic and subjective/behavioral symptoms of anxiety (see Special Information). (see *DSM-IV* Criteria Appendix, p 329) **300.23 Social Phobia** This phobia involves a marked and persistent fear of one or more social or performance situations in which the person is exposed to unfamiliar people or to possible scrutiny by others. The person recognizes the fear is excessive or unreasonable. Avoidance of the situation leads to impaired functioning. (see *DSM-IV* Criteria Appendix, p 345) **300.29 Specific Phobia** Marked and persistent fear that is excessive or unreasonable, cued by the presence or anticipation of a specific object or situation. Exposure to the phobic stimulus provokes an immediate anxiety response. In individuals under 18 years, the duration is at least 6 months. The anxiety associated with the object/situation is not better accounted for by another mental disorder.	**Infancy** Rarely diagnosed in infancy. During the second year of life, fears and distress occurring in situations not ordinarily associated with expected anxiety that is not amenable to traditional soothing and has an irrational quality about it may suggest a disorder. The fears are, for example, intense or phobic reactions to cartoons or clowns, or excessive fear concerning parts of the house (e.g., attic or basement). **Early Childhood** Rarely diagnosed in this age group. In children, these disorders may be expressed by crying, tantrums, freezing, or clinging, or staying close to a familiar person. Young children may appear excessively timid in unfamiliar social settings, shrink from contact with others, refuse to participate in group play, typically stay on the periphery of social activities, and attempt to remain close to familiar adults to the extent that family life is disrupted. **Middle Childhood and Adolescence** Symptoms in middle childhood and adolescence generally include the physiologic symptoms associated with anxiety (restlessness, sweating, tension) (see Pain/Somatic Complaints cluster, p 173) and avoidance behaviors such as refusal to attend school and lack of participation in school, decline in classroom performance or social functions. In addition, an increase in worries and sleep disturbances are present.

SPECIAL INFORMATION
Generalized anxiety disorder has subsumed the *DSM-III-R* diagnosis of overanxious disorder. Severe apprehension about performance may lead to refusal to attend school. This must be distinguished from other causes of refusal, including realistically aversive conditions at school (e.g., the child is threatened or harassed), learning disabilities (see Academic Skills cluster, p 69), separation anxiety disorder (see below), truancy (the child is not anxious about performance or separation), and depression (see Sadness and Related Symptoms cluster, p 153). To make these diagnoses in children, there must be evidence of capacity for social relationships with adults. Because of the early onset and chronic course of the disorder, impairment in children tends to take the form of failure to achieve an expected level of functioning rather than a decline from optimal functioning. Children with generalized anxiety disorder may be overly conforming, perfectionistic, and unsure of themselves and tend to redo tasks because of being zealous in seeking approval and requiring excessive reassurance about their performance and other worries.

DISORDER	COMMON DEVELOPMENTAL PRESENTATIONS
309.21 Separation Anxiety Disorder Developmentally inappropriate and excessive anxiety concerning separation from home or from those to whom the individual is attached. (see *DSM-IV* Criteria Appendix, p 341)	**Infancy** Not relevant at disorder level. **Early and Middle Childhood** When separated from attachment figures, children may exhibit social withdrawal, apathy, sadness, difficulty concentrating on work or play. They may have fears of animals, monsters, the dark, muggers, kidnappers, burglars, car accidents; concerns about death and dying are common. When alone, young children may report unusual perceptual experiences (e.g., seeing people peering into their room). **Adolescence** Adolescents with this disorder may deny feeling anxiety about separation; however, it may be reflected in their limited independent activity and reluctance to leave home.
300.01 Panic Disorder This disorder involves recurrent unexpected (uncued) panic attacks. Apprehension and anxiety about the attacks or a significant change in behavior related to the attack persists for at least 1 month. A panic attack is a discrete episode of intense fear or discomfort with sudden onset combining the following psychological symptoms — a sense of impending doom, fear of going crazy, and feelings of unreality — with somatic symptoms such as shortness of breath/dyspnea, palpitations/tachycardia, sweating, choking, chest pain, nausea, dizziness, paresthesia. (see *DSM-IV* Criteria Appendix, p 336)	**Infancy** Not relevant at disorder level. **Early Childhood** In children, these disorders may be expressed by crying, tantrums, freezing, clinging, or staying close to a familiar person during a panic attack. **Middle Childhood** Panic attacks may be manifested by symptoms such as tachycardia, shortness of breath, spreading chest pain, and extreme tension. **Adolescence** The symptoms are similar to those seen in an adult, such as the sense of impending doom, fear of going crazy, feelings of unreality and somatic symptoms such as shortness of breath, palpitations, sweating, choking, and chest pain.
	SPECIAL INFORMATION
	Separation anxiety disorder must be beyond what is expected for the child's developmental level to be coded as a disorder. In infancy, consider a developmental variation or anxiety problem rather than separation anxiety disorder. Worry about separation may take the form of worry about the health and safety of self or parents. Separation anxiety disorder may begin as early as preschool age and may occur at any time before age 18 years, but onset as late as adolescence is uncommon. Use early onset specifier if the onset of disorder is before 6 years. Children with separation anxiety disorder are often described as demanding, intrusive, and in need of constant attention, which may lead to parental frustration. Separation anxiety disorder is a common cause of refusal to attend school. Parental difficulty in separating from the child may contribute to the clinical problem (see Mental disorder of parent, p 46). A breakdown in the marital relationship (marital discord) and one parent's overinvolvement with the child is often seen (see p 44). Children with serious current or past medical problems (see Chronic and acute health conditions, pp 52 and 53) may be overprotected by parents and at greater risk for separation anxiety disorder. Parental illness and death may also increase risk.

SPECIAL INFORMATION, CONTINUED
Although panic attacks can be overwhelming, the social impairment in panic disorders is the result of secondary avoidance, rather than the attacks themselves. Panic attacks or panic symptoms can occur in a variety of anxiety problems or disorders, including specific phobia, social phobia, separation anxiety disorder, and posttraumatic stress disorder. Panic attacks in these disorders, however, are situationally bound, or cued; that is, they are triggered by specific contexts or environmental stimuli. Unexpected or uncued panic attacks must occur for a diagnosis of panic disorder. Major depressive disorder frequently (50% to 65%) occurs in individuals with panic disorder.

DISORDER	COMMON DEVELOPMENTAL PRESENTATIONS
309.81 Posttraumatic Stress Disorder (PTSD) PTSD occurs following exposure to an event that involved actual or threatened death or serious injury, or a threat to the physical integrity of self or others. The child or adolescent has symptoms in each of the following three areas for more than 1 month, causing significant distress or impairment of functioning: (1) persistent reexperiencing of the trauma, (2) avoidance of stimuli associated with the trauma and diminished general responsiveness, and (3) increased arousal or hypervigilance. In infancy, a numbing of responsiveness may also occur. (see *DSM-IV* Criteria Appendix, p 339) **308.3 Acute Stress Disorder** (see *DSM-IV* Criteria Appendix, p 311)	**Infancy** Rarely diagnosed but may take the form of extra fears or aggressive behaviors in response to stress. **Early Childhood, Middle Childhood, Adolescence** In children, distressing dreams of the event may, within several weeks, change into generalized nightmares of monsters, of rescuing others, or of threats to self or others. Reliving of the trauma may occur through repetitive play. Children may also exhibit various physical symptoms, such as stomachaches and headaches.
	SPECIAL INFORMATION
	PTSD follows exposure to acute or chronic stressors that involve actual or threatened death or serious injury to the child or others. The child must have reacted with intense fear, disorganized or agitated behavior, or helplessness. Stressors may be acute or chronic, single or multiple. PTSD may be chronic and associated with significant morbidity. Symptoms of repetitive trauma re-enacting play and a sense of a foreshortened future may persist after distress is no longer present. PTSD must be distinguished from normal bereavement. Bereavement is characterized by sadness and recurrent thoughts, but not by persistent impairment of functioning (see Sadness and Related Symptoms cluster, p 153). Consider sexual abuse/rape (p 45). Because it may be difficult for children to report diminished interest in significant activities and constriction of affect, these symptoms should be carefully evaluated with reports from parents and teachers. In children, the sense of a foreshortened future may be evidenced by the belief that life will be too short to include becoming an adult.

DIFFERENTIAL DIAGNOSIS	SPECIAL INFORMATION
General Medical Conditions Endocrine Hyperthyroidism Hypoglycemia Pheochromocytoma Others Mitral valve prolapse, especially when related to panic Acute bronchospasm	If a general medical condition is producing anxiety-like symptoms, the medical condition should be coded and **anxiety disorder due to a general medical condition** should be coded as **293.84.** If there is an overreaction to a medical condition consider adjustment disorder with anxious mood.
Substance-Related Anxiety Symptoms Stimulant medications ß-agonists Cocaine Phenylpropanolamine Withdrawal from central nervous system (CNS) depressants	Symptoms are produced by central nervous system stimulants and withdrawal from CNS depressants. If substance withdrawal is producing anxiety-like symptoms, the specific substance abuse problem should be coded, and substance-induced anxiety disorder should also be noted. If prescription medication (or withdrawal from medication) is causing anxiety symptoms, code substance-induced anxiety disorder and note the specific medication involved.
Mental Disorders 314.xx Attention-deficit/hyperactivity disorder (ADHD) 300.3 Obsessive-compulsive disorder 296.xx Major depressive disorder 300.4 Dysthymic disorder	Anxiety can be a manifestation of virtually every psychiatric syndrome. To be classified as an anxiety problem or disorder, anxiety must be the central feature of the disturbance.

COMMONLY COMORBID CONDITIONS	SPECIAL INFORMATION
Other Comorbid Mental Health Conditions Anxiety disorders are frequently comorbid with ADHD and depressive disorders.	If the child meets criteria for both an anxiety disorder and a depressive disorder or ADHD, both disorders should be coded. Multiple anxiety diagnoses are often present
Other General Medical Conditions Any serious medical condition may be associated with anxiety. Children may experience anxiety symptoms or reactive anxiety problems in relation to hospitalization and medical or surgical procedures. Mitral valve prolapse is associated with panic disorder.	Code medical diagnosis and anxiety symptoms or problem. Code mitral valve prolapse and panic disorder.

Presenting Complaints

sad/depressed

apathetic

loss of pleasure

agitation

sleep disturbance

appetite changes

decreased energy

decreased concentration

low self-esteem

crying

irritability

Definitions and Symptoms

Sadness, irritability, or a loss of interest in normally pleasurable activities is a common and normal response to disappointment, failure, or loss. Such mood changes only represent a problem if they persist more than a few days and if they represent intense distress or significantly impair the child's ability to function or relate to others at home, school, or play. It is recommended that assessment of suicidal ideation, plan, and intent be undertaken routinely when these symptoms are present. Children and adolescents may not present with sadness, but may report aches and pains, low energy, or moods such as apathy, irritability, or even anxiety. The mood disorders include major depressive disorder, dysthymic disorder, bipolar disorders, and cyclothymic disorder. To meet criteria for major depressive disorder, children must present with: 1) depressed or irritable mood, or 2) markedly diminished interest or pleasure in all, or almost all, activities. Bereavement is an intense grief response after a major loss (e.g., death of parent) and is usually a normal reaction involving mood and sleep or appetite changes. When bereavement symptoms persist for longer than 2 months or are characterized by marked functional impairment, morbid preoccupation with worthlessness or suicidal ideation, major depressive disorder can be diagnosed.

Approximately one third of teenagers with depression receive treatment. This is particularly problematic given the recurrent nature of depressive episodes, the possibility of suicide, and the heightened risk of greater frequency and severity of depressive disorders in adulthood for patients with early onset (before 20 years of age). Risk factors include depressed parent(s) (see Mental disorder of parent, p 46), a strong family history of depression, anxiety disorder, alcoholism, family and marital discord (see p 44), substance abuse (see Substance Use/Abuse cluster, p 135), uncertainty about sexual orientation, and a history of previous depressive episodes. The presence of suicidal ideation, a history of suicide attempt(s), or suicidal behavior among family members or friends should trigger a prompt and thorough evaluation of suicide potential (see Suicidal Thoughts or Behaviors cluster, p 165).

Epidemiology

Symptoms of depression are more prevalent in adolescence than in younger children and the rise may be due to a function of puberty rather than chronological age. Depressive disorders become more frequent during adolescence with a possible parallel shift in the sex ratio from a male preponderance before puberty to a female preponderance after puberty. Immediate grief reactions following bereavement tend to be milder and of a shorter duration in younger children compared with those in adolescence or adulthood. In the 14- to 18-year-old age group, the 1-year total incidence of depressive disorders is estimated to be 7.7%; most cases meet the criteria for a major depressive disorder. Prevalence and incidence rates are approximately twice as high for girls as for boys; this gender difference appears to emerge at about 12 to 13 years of age. Depression is 1½ to 3 times more common among first-degree biological relatives of persons with major depressive disorder than in the general population.

DEVELOPMENTAL VARIATION	COMMON DEVELOPMENTAL PRESENTATIONS
V65.49 Sadness Variation Transient depressive responses or mood changes to stress are normal in otherwise healthy populations. **V62.82 Bereavement** Sadness related to a major loss that typically persists for less than 2 months after the loss. However, the presence of certain symptoms that are not characteristic of a "normal" grief reaction may be helpful in differentiating bereavement from a major depressive disorder. These include guilt about things other than actions taken or not taken by the survivor at the time of death, thoughts of death, and morbid preoccupation with worthlessness.	**Infancy** The infant shows brief expressions of sadness, which normally first appear in the last quarter of the first year of life, manifest by crying, brief withdrawal, and transient anger. **Early Childhood** The child may have transient withdrawal and sad affect that may occur after losses and usually experiences bereavement due to the death of a parent or the loss of a pet or treasured object. **Middle Childhood** The child feels transient loss of self-esteem after experiencing failure and feels sadness with losses as in early childhood. **Adolescence** The adolescent's developmental presentations are similar to those of middle childhood but may also include fleeting thoughts of death. Bereavement includes loss of a boyfriend or girlfriend, friend, or best friend.

	SPECIAL INFORMATION

A normal process of bereavement occurs when a child experiences the death of or separation from someone (person or pet) loved by the child. There are normal age-specific responses as well as responses related to culture, temperament, the nature of the relationship between the child and the one the child is grieving, and the child's history of loss. While a child may manifest his or her grief response for a period of weeks to a couple of months, it is important to understand that the loss does not necessarily go away within that time frame. Most children will need to revisit the sadness at intervals (months or years) to continue to interpret the meaning of the loss to their life and to examine the usefulness of the coping mechanisms used to work through the sadness. A healthy mourning process requires that the child has a sense of reality about the death and access to incorporating this reality in an ongoing process of life. Unacknowledged, invalidated grief usually results in an unresolving process and leads to harmful behaviors toward self or others. Symptoms reflecting grief reaction may appear to be mild or transient, but care must be taken to observe subtle ways that unexpressed sadness may be exhibited.

Children in hospitals or institutions often experience some of the fears that accompany a death or separation. These fears may be demonstrated in actions that mimic normal grief responses.

PROBLEM	COMMON DEVELOPMENTAL PRESENTATIONS
V40.3 Sadness Problem Sadness or irritability that begins to include some symptoms of major depressive disorders in mild form. • depressed/irritable mood • diminished interest or pleasure • weight loss/gain, or failure to make expected weight gains • insomnia/hypersomnia • psychomotor agitation/retardation • fatigue or energy loss • feelings of worthlessness or excessive or inappropriate guilt • diminished ability to think/concentrate However, the behaviors are not sufficiently intense to qualify for a depressive disorder. These symptoms should be more than transient and have a mild impact on the child's functioning. Bereavement that continues beyond 2 months may also be a problem.	**Infancy** The infant may experience some developmental regressions, fearfulness, anorexia, failure to thrive, sleep disturbances, social withdrawal, irritability, and increased dependency, which are responsive to extra efforts at soothing and engagement by primary caretakers. **Early Childhood** The child may experience similar symptoms as in infancy, but sad affect may be more apparent. In addition, temper tantrums may increase in number and severity, and physical symptoms such as constipation, secondary enuresis (see Day/Nighttime Wetting Problems cluster, p 215), encopresis (see Soiling Problems cluster, p 209), and nightmares may be present. **Middle Childhood** The child may experience some sadness that results in brief suicidal ideation with no clear plan of suicide, some apathy, boredom, low self-esteem, and unexplained physical symptoms such as headaches and abdominal pain (see Pain/Somatic Complaints cluster, p 173). **Adolescence** Some disinterest in school work, decrease in motivation, and daydreaming in class may begin to lead to deterioration of school work. Hesitancy in attending school, apathy, and boredom may occur.

SPECIAL INFORMATION
Sadness is experienced by some children beyond the level of a normal developmental variation when the emotional or physiologic symptoms begin to interfere with effective social interactions, family functioning, or school performance. These periods of sadness may be brief or prolonged depending on the precipitating event and temperament of the child. Reassurance and monitoring is often needed at this level. If the sad behaviors are more severe, consider major depressive disorders. The potential for suicide in grieving children is higher. Evaluation of suicidal risk should be part of a grief workup for all patients expressing profound sadness or confusion or demonstrating destructive behaviors toward themselves or others. Behavioral symptoms resulting from bereavement that persist beyond 2 months after the loss require evaluation and intervention. Depressed parents or a strong family history of depression or alcoholism (see Mental disorder of parent, p 46) puts youth at very high risk for depressive problems and disorders. Family and marital discord, p 44, exacerbates risk. Suicidal ideation should be assessed (see Suicidal Thoughts or Behaviors cluster, p 165). Lying, stealing, suicidal thoughts (see Suicidal Thoughts or Behaviors cluster, p 165), and promiscuity may be present. Physical symptoms may include recurrent headaches, chronic fatigue, and abdominal pain (see Pain/Somatic Complaints cluster, p 173).

DISORDER	COMMON DEVELOPMENTAL PRESENTATIONS
296.2x, 296.3x Major Depressive Disorder Significant distress or impairment is manifested by five of the nine criteria listed below, occurring nearly every day for 2 weeks. These symptoms must represent a change from previous functioning and that either depressed or irritable mood or diminished interest or pleasure must be present to make the diagnosis. • depressed/irritable • diminished interest or pleasure • weight loss/gain • insomnia/hypersomnia • psychomotor agitation/retardation • fatigue or energy loss • feelings of worthlessness • diminished ability to think/concentrate • recurrent thoughts of death and suicidal ideation (see *DSM-IV* Criteria Appendix, p 332)	**Infancy** True major depressive disorders are difficult to diagnose in infancy. However, the reaction of some infants in response to the environmental cause is characterized by persistent apathy, despondency (often associated with the loss of a caregiver or an unavailable [e.g., severely depressed] caregiver), nonorganic failure-to-thrive (often associated with apathy, excessive withdrawal), and sleep difficulties. These reactions, in contrast to the "problem" level, require significant interventions. **Early Childhood** This situation in early childhood is similar to infancy. **Middle Childhood** The child frequently experiences chronic fatigue, irritability, depressed mood, guilt, somatic complaints, and is socially withdrawn (see Pain/Somatic Complaints cluster, p 173). Psychotic symptoms (hallucinations or delusions) may be present. **Adolescence** The adolescent may display psychomotor retardation or have hypersomnia. Delusions or hallucinations are not uncommon (but not part of the specific symptoms of the disorder).

SPECIAL INFORMATION
Depressed parents or a strong family history of depression or alcoholism puts youth at very high risk for depressive disorder (see Mental disorder of parent, p 46). Risk is increased by family and marital discord, p 44), substance abuse by the patient (see Substance Use/Abuse cluster, p 135), and a history of depressive episodes. Suicidal ideation should be routinely assessed. Sex distribution of the disorder is equivalent until adolescence, when females are twice as likely as males to have a depressive disorder. Culture can influence the experience and communication of symptoms of depression, (e.g., in some cultures, depression tends to be expressed largely in somatic terms rather than with sadness or guilt). Complaints of "nerves" and headaches (in Latino and Mediterranean cultures), of weakness, tiredness, or "imbalance" (in Chinese and Asian cultures), of problems of the "heart" (in Middle Eastern cultures), or of being "heartbroken" (among Hopis) may express the depressive experience. Subsequent depressive episodes are common. Bereavement typically improves steadily without specific treatment. If significant impairment or distress is still present after 2 months following the acute loss or death of a loved one, or if certain symptoms that are not characteristic of a "normal" grief reaction are present (e.g., marked functional impairment, morbid preoccupation with worthlessness, suicidal ideation, psychotic symptoms, or psychomotor retardation), consider diagnosis and treatment of major depressive disorder.

DISORDER	COMMON DEVELOPMENTAL PRESENTATIONS
300.4 Dysthymic Disorder The symptoms of dysthymic disorder are less severe or disabling than those of major depressive disorder but more persistent. Depressed/irritable mood for most of the day, for more days than not (either by subjective account or observations of others) for at least 1 year. Also the presence, while depressed/irritable, of two (or more) of the following: • poor appetite/overeating • insomnia/hypersomnia • low energy or fatigue • poor concentration/difficulty making decisions • feelings of hopelessness (see *DSM-IV* Criteria Appendix, p 326)	**Infancy** Not diagnosed. **Early Childhood** Rarely diagnosed. **Middle Childhood and Adolescence** Commonly experience feelings of inadequacy, loss of interest/pleasure, social withdrawal, guilt/brooding, irritability or excessive anger, decreased activity/productivity. May experience sleep/appetite/weight changes and psychomotor symptoms. Low self-esteem is common.

	SPECIAL INFORMATION
309.0 Adjustment Disorder With Depressed Mood (see *DSM-IV* Criteria Appendix, p 312) **311 Depressive Disorder, Not Otherwise Specified**	Because of the chronic nature of the disorder, the child may not develop adequate social skills. The child is at risk for episodes of major depression.

DISORDER	COMMON DEVELOPMENTAL PRESENTATIONS
296.0x Bipolar I Disorder, With Single Manic Episode (see *DSM-IV* Criteria Appendix, p 319) **296.89 Bipolar II Disorder, Recurrent Major Depressive Episodes With Hypomanic Episodes** Includes presence (or history) of one or more major depressive episodes, presence of at least one hypomanic episode, there has never been a manic episode (similar to manic episodes but only need to be present for 4 or more days and are not severe enough to cause marked impairment in function) or a mixed episode. The symptoms are not better accounted for by schizoaffective disorder, schizophrenia, delusional disorder, or psychotic disorder. The symptoms cause clinically significant distress or impairment in social, occupational, or other important areas of functioning.	**Infancy** Not diagnosed. **Early Childhood** Rarely diagnosed. **Middle Childhood** The beginning symptoms as described for adolescents start to appear. **Adolescence** During manic episodes, adolescents may wear flamboyant clothing, distribute gifts or money, and drive recklessly. They display inflated self-esteem, a decreased need for sleep, pressure to keep talking, flights of ideas, distractibility, unrestrained buying sprees, sexual indiscretion, school truancy and failure, antisocial behavior, and illicit drug experimentation.

SPECIAL INFORMATION

Substance abuse is commonly associated with bipolar disorder (see Substance Use/Abuse cluster, p 135).

Stimulant abuse and certain symptoms of attention-deficit/hyperactivity disorder may mimic a manic episode (see Hyperactive/Impulsive Behaviors cluster, p 93).

Manic episodes in children and adolescents can include psychotic features and may be associated with school truancy, antisocial behavior (see Secretive Antisocial Behaviors cluster, p 127), school failure, or illicit drug experimentation. Longstanding behavior problems often precede the first manic episode.

One or more manic episodes (a distinct period of an abnormally and persistently elevated and expansive or irritable mood lasting at least 1 week if not treated) frequently occur with one or more major depressive episodes. The symptoms are not better accounted for by other severe mental disorders (e.g., schizoaffective, schizophrenegenic, delusional, or psychotic disorders). The symptoms cause mild impairment in functioning in usual social activities and relationships with others.

DIFFERENTIAL DIAGNOSIS	SPECIAL INFORMATION
General Medical Conditions — Examples include: Endocrine abnormalities, e.g., thyroid disorders Malignancies Malnutrition Mononucleosis Chronic fatigue syndrome Neurologic disorders Autoimmune disorders Metabolic disorders	Almost any medical condition can cause fatigue, loss of energy, insomnia, changes in appetite, and other symptoms of depression. If a general medical condition is producing mood disturbance problems, the medical condition should be coded, and mood disorder due to a general medical condition should be coded as **293.83.**
Substances — Examples include: Alcohol abuse Drug abuse Prescription drug side effects (reserpine, glucocorticoids, anabolic steroids) Over-the-counter drugs containing synthetic narcotics	Code substance-induced mood disorder.
Mental Disorders 309.0 Adjustment disorder with depressed mood 314.xx Attention-deficit/hyperactivity disorder 300.82 Somatization disorder 293.83 Mood disorders due to a general medical condition	

COMMONLY COMORBID CONDITIONS	SPECIAL INFORMATION
Other Comorbid Mental Health Conditions — Examples include: 300.3 Obsessive-compulsive disorder 307.80 Panic disorders 312.81 Conduct disorder childhood onset 312.82 Conduct disorder adolescent onset 313.81 Oppositional defiant disorder 305 Substance abuse disorder 314.xx Attention-deficit/hyperactivity disorder 295. Schizophrenia 299.00 Autistic disorder 307.1 Anorexia nervosa 307.51 Bulimia nervosa 300.02 Generalized anxiety disorder 309.81 Posttraumatic stress disorder 309.21 Separation anxiety disorder	In children, major depressive disorders occur more frequently in conjunction with other mental disorders (especially disruptive behavior and anxiety disorders, and attention-deficit/hyperactivity disorder).
Other General Medical Conditions that are acute, chronic, or disabling.	Especially prevalent in chronic conditions that significantly affect appearance or ability to engage in age-appropriate activities (e.g., diabetes, cystic fibrosis). If this occurs, code both conditions.

Presenting Complaints

rituals

obsessions

compulsions

Definition and Symptoms

Obsessions are recurrent and persistent thoughts, impulses, or images that are intrusive, inappropriate, and cause marked anxiety or distress. The thoughts, impulses, or images are not simply excessive worry about real-life problems. The person attempts to ignore, suppress, or neutralize these obsessions with some other thought or action. Although adults recognize that the thoughts, impulses, or images are a product of their own minds, children, because they may lack sufficient cognitive awareness, may not be able to make this judgment. Common obsessions include repeated thoughts about contamination, doubts about behavior (having locked the door), and aggressive horrific impulses. Compulsions are repetitive behaviors or mental acts that the person feels driven to perform in response to an obsession, or according to rules that must be applied rigidly. The behaviors or mental acts are aimed at preventing or reducing distress or preventing some dreaded event or situation. Common compulsions include repeated hand washing, ordering, checking, and certain mental acts (e.g., counting, repeating words). Also common are "playful" compulsions of middle childhood such as not stepping "on a crack" in the sidewalk. Children generally do not request help for compulsions and obsessions. The problem is most often identified by parents, who bring the child in for treatment. Gradual declines in school work secondary to impaired ability to concentrate have been reported. Like adults, children are more prone to engage in rituals at home than in front of peers, teachers, or strangers.

Epidemiology

Recent community studies have estimated a lifetime prevalence of obsessive-compulsive disorder of 2.5% and 1-year prevalence of 1.5% to 2.1%. Onset in males tends to be earlier than in females. The disorder is equally common in males and females.

DEVELOPMENTAL VARIATION	COMMON DEVELOPMENTAL PRESENTATIONS
V65.49 Ritual Variation Rituals, obsessions, or compulsions that do not affect normal development.	**Infancy** The infant may need rigid bedtime rituals (necessary order of song, bottle, rocking). The infant needs a particular security object. Sometimes repetitions are related to mastery. The rituals are of short duration and do not interfere with normal day-to-day activities. **Early Childhood** The child has bedtime rituals or takes an interest in lining up toys and ordering things. The rituals are of short duration and do not interfere with normal day-to-day activities. **Middle Childhood** The child engages in repetitive habits (hair twirling) and game rituals. **Adolescence** The adolescent grooms excessively and has particular exercise patterns but these do not interfere with normal daily activities and the adolescent is not rigid in the routine.

	SPECIAL INFORMATION
	These behaviors may be normative at certain stages but can also cause concern for parents.

PROBLEM	COMMON DEVELOPMENTAL PRESENTATIONS
V40.3 Ritual, Obsessive, Compulsive Problem Rituals, obsessions, or compulsions that are unwanted by the child and sometimes restrict activities.	**Infancy and Early Childhood** Develops perseverative activities with rituals or repetitive order and becomes agitated with changes. **Middle Childhood** In middle childhood, the child may develop some obsessions or compulsions such as repeatedly counting, washing hands, twirling hair, preoccupations with even and odd numbers (insists on counting by two's, changes place in line to avoid odd numbers), or with rearranging (insists on ordering from small to large or grouping certain colors) but retains some flexibility so that these only interfere with activities sometimes. **Adolescence** In adolescence, there may be a preoccupation with grooming compulsions, hair twirling and pulling, nail biting, and rereading and rewriting homework. These will sometimes interfere with activities.

DISORDER	COMMON DEVELOPMENTAL PRESENTATIONS
300.3 Obsessive-Compulsive Disorder The obsessions and/or compulsions interfere with functioning, cause marked distress, or occupy more than 1 hour a day. (see *DSM-IV* Criteria Appendix, p 334) **300.00 Anxiety Disorder, Not Otherwise Specified**	**Infancy** Rarely presents at this age. **Early Childhood** The child evidences a higher degree of compulsive and ritualistic behavior, from holding onto certain objects, watching certain videotapes, or lining up toys in certain sequences. These rigidities are less responsive to soothing and interaction than at the problem level. When these ritualistic behaviors are associated with problems in relating and communicating (see Social Interaction Behaviors cluster, p 277). **Middle Childhood and Adolescence** The child presents with obsessions and compulsions such as repetitive hand washing, ordering, checking, counting, repeating words silently, repetitive praying. The obsessions or compulsions interfere with listening or attending in class and frequently grades worsen because the child cannot sit still during tests or lectures. The child may fear harming himself or herself or others if compulsion is not performed and has problems with task completion.
	SPECIAL INFORMATION
	The child may be reluctant to talk about the condition; parental report may be the only reliable history. Sexuality may be the underlying concern in certain cases (see Sexual Development Behaviors cluster, p 261). Children are more prone to engage in rituals at home than in front of peers, teachers, or strangers. Although obsessive-compulsive disorder usually presents in adolescence or early adulthood, it may begin in childhood. For the most part onset is gradual, but acute onset has been noted in some cases.

DIFFERENTIAL DIAGNOSIS	SPECIAL INFORMATION
General Medical Conditions No specific conditions.	
Substances Cocaine or amphetamine abuse can cause repetitive, ritualistic behaviors. Substance-induced anxiety disorder (refer to *DSM-IV* Criteria Appendix, p 349, for specific substance codes)	
Mental Disorders 299.00　Autistic disorder 317,　　Mental retardation 318.x, 319 307.1　　Anorexia nervosa 296.xx　Major depressive disorder 293.84　Anxiety disorder due to a 　　　　　general medical condition 300.02　Generalized anxiety disorder 300.29　Specific phobia 300.23　Social phobia 300.7　　Body dysmorphic disorder 300.7　　Hypochondriasis 297.1　　Delusional disorder 312.39　Trichotillomania	

COMMONLY COMORBID CONDITIONS	SPECIAL INFORMATION
Other Comorbid Mental Health Conditions — Examples include: 301.23　Tourette's disorder 313.23　Selective mutism 314.xx　Attention-deficit/hyperactivity 　　　　　disorder 296.2x,　Major depressive disorder 296.3x 300.09　Generalized anxiety disorder 307.1　　Anorexia nervosa 301.4　　Obsessive-compulsive 　　　　　personality disorder 307.51　Bulimia nervosa	There is a high incidence of obsessive-compulsive disorder in individuals with Tourette's disorder, with estimates ranging from approximately 35% to 50%. The incidence of Tourette's disorder in obsessive-compulsive disorder is lower, with estimates ranging between 5% and 7%. Treating the associated psychiatric disorder may be useful in decreasing obsessive-compulsive symptoms.
Other General Medical Conditions Dermatological problems	Dermatological problems caused by excessive washing with water or caustic cleaning agents may be observed.

Presenting Complaints

thinking that life is not worth living
passive or active wish to die
thinking about hurting oneself
intending to hurt oneself
having a plan to hurt oneself
history of attempting suicide

Definition and Symptoms

Suicidal behavior includes a child's stated or unstated thoughts about causing intentional self-injury or death (suicidal ideation) and acts that cause intentional self-injury (suicide attempts) or death (suicide). Intent to cause harm to oneself is an essential ingredient in defining suicidal behavior. Intent may be explicit and strong, or it may be ambiguous and not well defined. Three categories of problems should prompt the primary care physician to probe further regarding suicidal risk: 1) psychiatric problems, depression (see Sadness and Related Symptoms cluster, p 153), substance abuse (see Substance Use/Abuse cluster, p 135), conduct problems (see Aggressive/Oppositional Behaviors cluster, p 119), psychosis, past suicidal threats or behavior; 2) poor social adjustment (school failure, legal problems, social isolation, interpersonal conflict); and 3) family/environmental problems (interpersonal loss, abuse or neglect, runaway or homeless, family history of psychiatric disorder or suicide, exposure to suicide [see Environmental Situations Defined, p 31]). It is important for the physician to ask directly about suicidal ideation and plans. Routine clinical inquiry will not elicit these thoughts and concerns from an individual. Those with a specific plan and/or intent or specific risk factors should be considered at most risk. Among patients who present to primary care physicians, the following are indicative of high risk for suicidal behavior: 1) presenting complaint that involves a mental health problem; 2) recent history of physical or sexual assault; 3) history of suicidal behavior; and 4) those exposed to suicide through school or media. Among those with chronic illness, suicidal ideation and behavior may be more common in those with diabetes and epilepsy.

Epidemiology

Suicide is the second leading cause of death among older adolescents. Between 12% and 25% of primary school and high school children have some form of suicidal ideation. The rate of suicide has tripled since the 1950s, which may be due to the increased availability and use of alcohol and firearms among youth. In addition, the rate of suicidal behavior has become much more common to the extent that 4% of high school students have made an attempt within the previous 12 months and 8% have made an attempt in their lifetime. Only one in eight suicide attempts is brought to the attention of a medical professional.

Among children and adolescents, the suicide rate and the rate of attempted suicide increase with age. The rate of completed suicide is much higher among males; however, the rate of attempted suicides is much higher among females. This higher rate of completed suicides among males is thought to be attributed to the more violent means utilized by males. The suicide rate is also much higher among whites than blacks, although the rates in both groups have increased. Native Americans have been reported to have a particularly high suicide rate. Socioeconomic status in general does not affect the rate of suicide, but a low status appears to be associated with higher rates of attempts. Uncertainty about sexual orientation also increases risk for suicide.

DEVELOPMENTAL VARIATION	COMMON DEVELOPMENTAL PRESENTATIONS
V65.49 Thoughts of Death Variation Anxiety about death in early childhood. Focus on death in middle childhood or adolescence.	**Infancy** Not relevant at this age. **Early Childhood** In early childhood anxiety about dying may be present. **Middle Childhood** Anxiety about dying may occur in middle childhood, especially after a death in the family. **Adolescence** Some interest with death and morbid ideation may be manifest by a preference for black clothing and an interest in the occult. If this becomes increased to a point of preoccupation, a problem or a serious ideation should be considered.

PROBLEM	COMMON DEVELOPMENTAL PRESENTATIONS
V40.2 Thoughts of Death Problem The child has thoughts of or a preoccupation with his or her own death. If the child has thoughts of suicide, consider suicidal ideation and attempts (next page).	**Infancy** Unable to assess. **Early and Middle Childhood** The child may express a wish to die through discussion or play. This often follows significant punishment or disappointment. **Adolescence** The adolescent may express nonspecific ideation related to suicide.
	SPECIAL INFORMATION
	Between 12% and 25% of primary school and high school children have some form of suicidal ideation. Those with a specific plan or specific risk factors should be considered at most risk.

DISORDER	COMMON DEVELOPMENTAL PRESENTATIONS
313.89 Suicidal Ideation and Attempts The child has thoughts about causing intentional self-harm acts that cause intentional self-harm or death. This code represents an unspecified mental disorder. It is to be used when no other condition is identified.	**Infancy** Unable to assess. **Early Childhood** The child expresses a wish and intent to die either verbally or by actions. **Middle Childhood** The child plans and enacts self-injurious acts with a variety of potentially lethal methods. **Adolescence** The adolescent frequently shows a strong wish to die and may carefully plan and carry out a suicide.

SPECIAL INFORMATION

A youngster's understanding that death is final is not an essential ingredient in considering a child or adolescent to be suicidal. However, very young children, such as preschoolers who do not appreciate the finality of death, can be considered to be suicidal if they wish to carry out a self-destructive act with the goal of causing death. Such behavior in preschoolers is often associated with physical or sexual abuse (see p 45).

Prepubertal children may be protected against suicide by their cognitive immaturity and limited access to more lethal methods that may prevent them from planning and executing a lethal suicide attempt despite suicidal impulses.

The suicide rate and rate of attempted suicide increase with age and with the presence of alcohol and other drug use. Psychotic symptoms, including hallucinations, increase risk as well.

Because of societal pressures, some homosexual youth are at increased risk for suicide attempts (see Gender Identity Issues cluster, p 255).

In cases of attempted suicide that are carefully planned, adolescents may leave a note, choose a clearly lethal method, and state their intent prior to the actual suicide. In contrast, most suicide attempts in adolescence are impulsive, sometimes with little threat to the patient's life. The motivation for most attempts appears to be a wish to gain attention and/or help, escape a difficult situation, or express anger or love. However, irrespective of motivation, all suicide attempts require careful evaluation and all patients with active intent to harm themselves should have a thorough psychiatric evaluation.

Although suicidal ideation and attempts is not a disorder diagnosis, more extensive evaluation may identify other mental conditions (e.g., major depressive disorder).

DIFFERENTIAL DIAGNOSIS	SPECIAL INFORMATION
General Medical Conditions Not relevant.	Suicidal ideation can occur simultaneously with any general medical condition.
Substances	Intoxication can exacerbate suicidal behaviors or ideation and should be considered a significant risk factor.
Mental Disorders Not relevant.	No medical disorders would be coded in place of suicidal ideation but do frequently occur simultaneously as described under Other Comorbid Mental Health Conditions.

COMMONLY COMORBID CONDITIONS	SPECIAL INFORMATION
Other Comorbid Mental Health Conditions — Examples include: **296.2x,** Major depressive disorder **296.3x** **309.xx** Adjustment disorder **305** Substance abuse disorder **295.xx** Schizophrenia **296.xx** Bipolar disorders **V62.82** Bereavement **301.83** Borderline personality disorder	Individuals with borderline personality disorder display recurrent suicidal behavior, gestures or threats, or self-mutilating behavior. Completed suicide occurs in 8% to 10% of such individuals, and self-mutilating acts (e.g., cutting or burning) and suicide threats and attempts are very common. Recurrent suicidality is often the reason that these individuals present for help. Only consider borderline personality disorder in later adolescence and early adulthood when a personality disorder can be diagnosed more reliably. Mental disorders can frequently be associated with suicidal ideations, these include depression (see Sadness and Related Symptoms cluster, p 153) or conduct problems (see Aggressive/Oppositional Behaviors cluster, p 119).
Other General Medical Conditions Chronic illness may predispose to suicidal ideation and suicide attempts (based on specific studies with diabetes and epilepsy).	

SOMATIC AND SLEEP BEHAVIORS

PAIN/SOMATIC COMPLAINTS

EXCESSIVE DAYTIME SLEEPINESS

SLEEPLESSNESS

NOCTURNAL AROUSALS

Presenting Complaints

abdominal pain

headaches

fatigue

limb pain

chest pain

back pain

worry about health or appearance

Definitions and Symptoms

Pain is an unpleasant sensory and emotional experience associated with actual or potential tissue damage, or described in terms of such damage. It may be acute or chronic. Pain is always subjective. Enormous individual differences in response to painful stimuli exist. The pain stimulus is interpreted based on the context or meaning of the pain to the individual, as well as the individual's psychological state, culture, previous experience, and a host of other psychosocial variables. As a result, the same noxious stimulus may cause different amounts of pain in different individuals based on personal characteristics. A relation between the amount of pain an individual reports and any associated tissue damage does not necessarily exist.

Infants and young children tend to be more acutely reactive to painful stimuli. This reaction tends to decrease as children age and are cognitively more capable of understanding the internal workings of the body and the notion that short-term discomfort may have long-term benefit. With chronic or recurrent pains, children may react by withdrawal, regression, or heightened anxiety depending on age and temperament. Family factors, particularly beliefs related to pain and illness, are important issues to consider in assessing children in pain.

Somatization refers to the occurrence of one or more physical complaints for which appropriate medical evaluation reveals no explanatory physical pathology or pathophysiologic mechanism or, when physical pathology is present, the physical complaints resulting in impairment are grossly in excess of what would be expected from the known physical findings.

Reporting pain and somatic complaints is quite common in childhood and adolescence. Such complaints may occur in the context of physical disease but may also occur in the apparent absence of physical disease or a known pathophysiologic process. Pain and somatic symptoms become problematic when, regardless of etiology, they become a dominant force in the child's life and impede normal development or interfere with functioning. These complaints may have multiple origins and should not be understood simply in terms of the presence of general medical pathology.

Patients with medically unexplained physical symptoms often have associated psychiatric symptoms, particularly symptoms of anxiety or depression. Separation fears may be particularly common in patients with recurrent pain syndromes. Such patients may be at risk for unnecessary medical investigations and treatments that can prove costly and potentially dangerous. They may use health care services excessively. There are seven types of somatoform disorders in *DSM-IV*: Somatization disorder, undifferentiated somatoform disorder, conversion disorder, pain disorder, hypochondriasis, body dysmorphic disorder, and somatoform disorder not otherwise specified. Hypochondriasis, the preoccupation with the fear of having, or the idea that one has, a serious disease based on the person's misinterpretation of bodily symptoms or body functions; and body dysmorphic disorder, the preoccupation with an imagined or exaggerated defect in physical appearance, will not be discussed in this section. See the *DSM-IV* Criteria Appendix, beginning on p 311, for the diagnostic criteria for these disorders.

Epidemiology

Studies have reported wide variability in lifetime prevalence rates of somatization disorder, ranging from 0.2% to 2% among women and less than 0.2% in men. Prevalence rates of conversion disorder range from 1% to 3% in outpatient referrals to mental health clinics. Recurrent complaints of pain are prevalent in the pediatric population, with some clinicians diagnosing a recurrent pain syndrome when the pain occurs at least three times within a 3-month period. Headache appears to be the most commonly reported of painful somatic symptoms, followed by recurrent abdominal pain, limb pain, and chest pain. Other commonly reported complaints include fatigue, dizziness, and gastrointestinal complaints such as nausea and vomiting. Pseudoneurologic symptoms such as pseudoseizures, medically unexplained gait abnormalities, and sensory abnormalities are actually relatively rare in community samples, though they may be more likely to be seen in tertiary care medical settings. Somatization may be polysymptomatic. Somatization disorder as described in adults is actually unusual in the pediatric age group.

DEVELOPMENTAL VARIATION	COMMON DEVELOPMENTAL PRESENTATIONS
V65.49 Somatic Complaint Variation Transient somatic complaints and discomfort that are associated with normal activity and growth and do not interfere with normal functioning.	**Infancy** The infant experiences transient gastrointestinal distress. **Early Childhood** The child experiences transient pain, experiences fatigue, has gastrointestinal distress, acquires minor bruises during play. These are not repetitive and do not interfere with a child's ability to function. **Middle Childhood** The child has transient aches and pains associated with normal activity and exertion, "growing pains," feels muscle strain, experiences transient fatigue, headaches, or gastrointestinal distress. These occur infrequently and do not interfere with the child's ability to function. **Adolescence** The adolescent has normal pains associated with female menstrual cycle and pubertal changes, and has other transient aches and pains accompanied by worry. These occur infrequently and do not impair the adolescent's ability to function.
	SPECIAL INFORMATION
	Pain is subjective; enormous individual variation exists. The intensity, duration, and frequency of pain, change in its level, and the context in which it occurs need to be assessed. The peak age for stomachaches is 9 years. The peak age for headaches is 12 years. Prior to puberty, no gender differences exist in the number of somatic complaints; females report more somatic complaints after puberty.

PROBLEM	COMMON DEVELOPMENTAL PRESENTATIONS
V40.3 Somatic Complaints Problem One or more physical complaints that cause some distress or functional impairment (e.g., in physical, social, or school activities) are considered a problem. The symptoms are not associated with a general medical condition or the general medical condition is not sufficient to explain the intensity or breadth of the symptoms. The symptoms are not sufficiently intense to qualify for a somatoform disorder.	**Infancy** The infant has more intense gastrointestinal distress interfering, to some degree, with feeding and sleep. **Early Childhood** The child complains about physical symptoms and sometimes avoids or refuses to undertake age-appropriate activities because of the symptoms. **Middle Childhood** The child complains about physical symptoms and sometimes avoids or refuses to undertake expected activities. **Adolescence** The adolescent has similar problems described for middle childhood and may use substances to self-medicate.

SPECIAL INFORMATION

Reports of somatic symptoms or pain should always first be evaluated for underlying general medical causes. Pain that is expected is often less extreme than pain from unexpected sources. Affective states (see Sadness and Related Symptoms cluster, p 153) are often associated with increased pain perception or somatic complaints. Multiple somatic complaints in children may be associated with parental reinforcement of illness behavior in the child.

In addition to somatic complaints, the child experiences emotional distress (see Anxious Symptoms cluster, p 145), is withdrawn (see Sadness and Related Symptoms cluster, p 153), has academic difficulties, refuses to attend school, is irritable, displays aggressive behaviors, and experiences recurrent pain syndromes.

DISORDER	COMMON DEVELOPMENTAL PRESENTATIONS

300.82 Undifferentiated Somatoform Disorder

One or more physical complaints (e.g., fatigue, loss of appetite, gastrointestinal or urinary complaints) that cause clinically significant distress or impairment in social, occupational, or other important areas of functioning, and persist for at least 6 months. The disturbance is not better accounted for by another mental disorder (e.g., mood disorder, anxiety disorder, sleep disorder, psychotic disorder). The symptoms are not intentionally produced or feigned. The symptoms cannot be fully explained by a general medical condition or the direct effects of a substance. If a general medical condition is present, the physical complaints or resulting impairment is in excess of what would be expected given the history, physical examination, or lab findings.

(see *DSM-IV* Criteria Appendix, p 350)

300.82 Somatoform Disorder

A history of physical complaints before age 30 years occurring over several years and resulting in treatment being sought or significant impairment. It needs to include four pain symptoms, two gastrointestinal symptoms, one sexual symptom, and one pseudoneurologic symptom. The symptoms cannot be fully explained by a known general medical condition or substance or are in excess of what needs to be expected.

307.80 Pain Disorder

Pain in one or more anatomical sites is the predominant focus of the clinical presentation and is of sufficient severity to warrant clinical attention. The pain causes clinically significant distress or impairment in school/occupational or other important areas of functioning. Psychological factors are judged to have an important role in the onset, severity, exacerbation, or maintenance of the pain. The pain is not intentionally produced or better accounted for by a mood, anxiety, or psychotic disorder. There are three types of pain disorder: **307.80** pain associated with psychological factors; **307.89** pain disorder associated with both psychological and a general medical condition; and pain disorder associated with a general medical condition.

(see *DSM-IV* Criteria Appendix, p 336)

COMMON DEVELOPMENTAL PRESENTATIONS

Infancy
Not relevant at this age.

Early Childhood
Rare at this age.

Middle Childhood
The child's symptoms do not usually meet the criteria for the full syndrome, although multiple and recurrent gastrointestinal, cardiopulmonary, or pain symptoms are not uncommon. Symptoms may be associated with significant academic or social problems because of school absences.

Adolescence
Symptoms for each of the three disorders usually begin during the teen years. Menstrual symptoms are common. The full syndrome may be diagnosed during late adolescence or early adulthood.

SPECIAL INFORMATION

A medical examination is needed to discover an organic basis for the pain. Pain may be associated with emotional distress. The onset or continuation of the pain may be temporarily associated with the psychological stressor(s) or avoidance of something aversive. In other words, symptoms may result in secondary gains such as a reduction of stress/academic pressures or family conflict. Children may also have mild pain syndrome that intensifies due to the secondary gains inadvertently achieved. These symptoms may be associated with frequent physician visits and unnecessary surgical interventions.

DISORDER, CONTINUED	COMMON DEVELOPMENTAL PRESENTATIONS
300.11 Conversion Disorder One or more symptoms or deficits affecting voluntary motor or sensory function that suggest a neurological or other general medical condition. Psychological factors are judged to be associated with the symptoms or deficit because the initiation or exacerbation of the symptom or deficit is preceded by conflicts or other stressors (see Environmental Situations Defined, p 31). The symptom or deficit cannot be fully explained by a general medical condition or the direct effects of a substance. (see *DSM-IV* Criteria Appendix, p 323) **300.16 Factitious Disorder** The intentional production or feigning of physical or psychological signs or symptoms in order to assume the sick role in the absence of external incentives. **300.82 Somatoform Disorder, Not Otherwise Specified** (see *DSM-IV* Criteria Appendix, p 345) **300.19 Factitious Disorder, Not Otherwise Specified** (see *DSM-IV* Criteria Appendix, p 328)	

DIFFERENTIAL DIAGNOSIS	SPECIAL INFORMATION
General Medical Conditions — **Examples include:** Arthritis Inflammatory bowel disease Peptic ulcer disease Brain tumor Chronic constipation Urinary tract infection Sickling syndromes such as sickle cell anemia	Increase in previously controlled pain or symptoms may be attributed to the spread of disease.
Substances	Substance use (often prescribed) may begin in response to symptoms; substance abuse may produce additional symptoms. Many medications may cause patient discomfort. If the patient is taking specific medications, consult the *Physician's Desk Reference* for possible side effects.
Mental Disorders **295.xx** Schizophrenia **296.xx** Major depressive disorder **300.2** Generalized anxiety disorder **300.7** Hypochondriasis **300.7** Body dysmorphic disorder **309.xx** Adjustment disorder **V65.2** Malingering	Major depressive disorders, anxiety disorders, and adjustment disorders frequently include unexplained physical complaints. Undifferentiated somatoform disorder is not diagnosed if the symptoms are better accounted for by one of these disorders (see Sadness and Related Symptoms cluster, p 153, and Anxious Symptoms cluster, p 145). Somatoform disorders and symptoms need to be distinguished from symptoms that are intentionally produced or feigned, either by child or parent.

COMMONLY COMORBID CONDITIONS	SPECIAL INFORMATION
Other Comorbid Mental Health **Conditions — Examples include:** **296.xx** Major depressive disorder **300.4** Dysthymic disorder **300.02** Generalized anxiety disorder **300.01** Panic disorder without agoraphobia **300.3** Obsessive-compulsive disorder **305** Substance abuse disorder **309.21** Separation anxiety **301.xx** Personality disorders	Consider physical or sexual abuse (see p 45), pressure for academic performance, illness in other family members, and the death of other family members (see Sadness and Related Symptoms cluster, p 153).
Other General **Medical Conditions** Not relevant.	Somatization problems may begin with any acute or chronic medical condition and should be suspected if the symptoms continue too long or are overelaborated.

Presenting Complaints

falling asleep at inappropriate times/activities
    (school, social occasions)
difficulty in awakening in the morning
resumption of daytime naps
inattention/hyperactivity
behavioral problems
failure in school

Definitions and Symptoms

The symptoms of excessive sleepiness include a wide array of behaviors that result from inadequate duration of sleep relative to the child's needs or poor-quality sleep because of sleep disruption secondary to a primary medical problem such as sleep apnea, or neurologic problem such as seizures, circadian factors when the child is attempting to remain awake during the circadian sleep phase, or primary neurologic determined sleepiness as seen in narcolepsy or as a side effect of drug use.

Excessive sleepiness can be defined simply as an increased tendency to fall asleep or to exhibit self-stimulating behaviors in an attempt to remain awake and to counteract the increased sleepiness. An important consideration in defining excessive sleepiness is an understanding of the developmental changes in sleep consolidation, sleep duration, and daytime nap tendency over childhood and adolescence. Normally children are excellent sleepers and extremely alert during the day except for discrete, well-defined, regular naps. The total sleep need of children and adolescents varies considerably from child to child, but generally remains consistent for any individual child. The general trend is for total sleep in a 24-hour period to decrease from infancy to middle childhood.

After 6 months of age, most children will have a well consolidated nighttime sleep of 9 to 12 hours' duration and daytime sleep consolidated into one to three naps. Generally, naps are discontinued some time between the ages of 2 to 5 years, and thereafter all of the child's sleep is consolidated into a long nighttime sleep of 9 to 12 hours. After naps have been discontinued during childhood, it is unusual for them to resume without an obvious cause. For a child, consistently falling asleep during daytime activities such as school, work, while playing, except at nap time when there is an obvious explanation, is *not* normal, is cause for concern, and demands active investigation.

During middle adolescence, objective sleepiness increases and the circadian phase tends to shift to a later time. Sleep need during adolescence is stable or *increased* compared to sleep need during preadolescence, and self-imposed or social-induced chronic sleep deprivation is normal.

Narcolepsy is a neurologically based disorder of primary hypersomnolence which often begins in adolescence or young adulthood but may present during early or middle childhood. The symptoms of narcolepsy are caused by dyscontrol of the timing of rapid eye movement (REM) and non-REM sleep and intrusion of some or all of the REM phenomena during the daytime and/or beginning of the night. Symptoms include excessive sleepiness and one or more of the following: 1) cataplexy — sudden loss of muscle tone and deep tendon reflexes triggered by intense emotion; 2) language, anger, surprise; 3) hypnagogic hallucinations — dreams at sleep onset; and 4) sleep paralysis.

Recurrent hypersomnia (Kleine-Levin syndrome) is a rare disorder characterized by recurrent episodes of excessive sleepiness lasting days to weeks in intervals that occur weeks or months apart. It most often occurs in adolescent males and often has associated behavioral abnormalities including binge eating, hypersexuality, irritability, and aggression, but may occur at any age in either males or females and may not have associated behavioral problems.

Delayed sleep phase syndrome is a circadian disorder during which the major sleep time is delayed in relation to desired clock time resulting in symptoms of sleep onset insomnia and difficulty in awakening in the morning. If associated with sleep deprivation, excessive daytime sleepiness results.

Obstructive sleep apnea (OSA)/obstructive hypoventilation (OHV) are disorders caused by partial or complete collapse of the pharyngeal airway during sleep, causing snoring, increased difficulty in breathing, sleep fragmentation secondary to apnea, and gas exchange abnormalities with hypoxia and hypercarbia. Excessive sleepiness from OSA/OHV is most often seen during middle childhood and adolescence.

Epidemiology

Excessive sleepiness in the face of an adequate amount of sleep occurring during the proper circadian phase, where there is no sleep fragmentation or underlying medical/neurologic problem, is rare in infancy, early childhood, and middle childhood.

The prevalence of narcolepsy is estimated at 0.03% to 0.16% of the general population. The prevalence of delayed sleep phase during adolescence is highly variable, ranging up to 7%. Inadequate sleep is the most common cause of excessive sleepiness in childhood. It is almost universal among high school students who have an early school start time and/or late evening extracurricular or employment obligations.

Etiology

Excessive sleepiness is mediated by three primary factors: 1) previous sleep duration relative to sleep needs, 2) sleep quality, and 3) circadian factors. Sleep deprivation is cumulative, with continued sleep restriction resulting in persistent hypersomnia. Sleep quality is affected by the continuity of sleep and is degraded by any medical, neurologic, or environmental conditions that cause frequent arousals. Drugs that facilitate the action of GABA (an inhibitory neurotransmitter) generally increase sleepiness, and drugs that facilitate dopaminergic activity increase alertness.

DEVELOPMENTAL VARIATION	COMMON DEVELOPMENTAL PRESENTATIONS
V65.49 Excessive Sleepiness Variation The amount of sleep an individual child needs varies greatly, although the child's need relative to the norm remains stable. While asleep, the child should appear peaceful, restful, and quiet, without snoring, evidence of respiratory difficulties, or frequent or prolonged arousals.	**Infancy** At birth most infants sleep 14 to 18 hours a day. Sleep does not have a circadian rhythm and is dispersed throughout 24 hours and superimposed on a 3- to 5-hour feeding schedule. By 6 months of age, the infant has developed a clear circadian rhythm. Nighttime sleep occurs at a predictable time and is generally well consolidated, although it may be punctuated by brief arousals for feeding with a rapid return to sleep for 8- to 14-hours' duration. Appropriate sleep onset associations and predictable routines are important in facilitating a rapid transition to sleep at bedtime and after normal nocturnal arousals. Nighttime sleep remains stable over infancy. Daytime sleep occurs during well-defined nap times. Although nap frequency and duration vary greatly among infants, the average nap schedule is three times a day at 6 months, twice a day at 12 months, and once a day after 18 months. The amount of daytime sleep is decreased during infancy as naps are discontinued. Total sleep time decreases during infancy because of decreasing daytime sleep. **Early Childhood** Nighttime sleep tends to remain stable at 8 to 12 hours from 6 months to 5 years of age. Generally, daytime naps are discontinued between 3 and 5 years. Total sleep time decreases as daytime naps are discontinued. Children are very alert between naps. **Middle Childhood** Nighttime sleep remains stable at 8 to 12 hours with an average of 11 hours. Daytime naps generally stop and children are at their peak alertness. Circadian factors have an important effect on sleepiness and conversely on alertness. A circadian increase in sleepiness occurs in the late afternoon (4 to 6 pm) independent of sleep duration and quality. This is the time of the siesta in cultures that have a bimodal sleep pattern. **Adolescence** Sleep needs do *not* decrease during adolescence and are probably very similar in any individual child to the amount of sleep needed during preadolescence (8 to 10 hours). Even if adolescents get the sleep they need, there is a modest increase in daytime sleepiness. A modest delay in sleep phase resulting in a later bedtime occurs commonly during adolescence. Increase in social, academic, and work demands often move bedtime later. Parents generally decrease their supervision of bedtime during early adolescence. All of these factors generally result in a later bedtime.
	SPECIAL INFORMATION
	Traveling across more than three time zones, especially in an eastward direction, is the most common cause of transient circadian problem that may result in difficulties at sleep onset, frequent nocturnal arousals, or excessive daytime sleepiness.

PROBLEM	COMMON DEVELOPMENTAL PRESENTATIONS
V40.3 Excessive Sleepiness Problem Excessive sleepiness becomes a problem when it has an impact on a child's ability to remain awake, attentive, and alert during the daytime. The most common cause of excessive sleepiness is simply an inadequate amount of sleep. It may also be caused by disruption of sleep because of frequent prolonged arousals or a delayed sleep phase. Code excessive sleepiness problem when the symptoms cause some impairment but are not of sufficient intensity to qualify for a primary hypersomnia disorder or narcolepsy diagnosis.	**Infancy and Early Childhood** An infant who is not provided with an adequate opportunity to sleep at night will make up for the loss during the day by taking frequent/long naps. **Middle Childhood and Adolescence** Sleep deprivation often starts becoming a factor in middle childhood and is almost universal during adolescence. Parents are generally much less involved in regulating bedtimes at this age. If the child is not arising spontaneously in the morning, if the child requires an alarm clock, a parent, or both to awaken him or her, it is an indication that more sleep is needed that night. The daytime consequences of excessive sleepiness may be falling asleep during activities such as school, riding the bus, or watching television. In a child with delayed sleep phase syndrome, sleep onset may be delayed presenting with the complaint of insomnia. This may foreshorten the nighttime sleep interval, contributing to sleep deprivation. On weekend nights the sleep time is often extended because of catch-up sleep; in which the arousal may be delayed until late morning or afternoon. Self-medication with caffeinated beverages and/or drugs may be used as a treatment for the sleepiness. Motivation to arise in the morning may play an important role, and refusal to attend school may be the underlying cause or a major contributor to the problem.
	SPECIAL INFORMATION
	After-school activities, part-time work, increased study demands, and early school starting times all tend to foreshorten nighttime sleep, contributing to chronic sleep deprivation.

DISORDER	COMMON DEVELOPMENTAL PRESENTATIONS
307.45 Circadian Rhythm Sleep Disorder — Delayed Sleep Phase Type A persistent or recurrent pattern of sleep disruption leading to excessive sleepiness or insomnia that is due to a mismatch between the sleep/wake schedule required by a person's environment and his or her circadian sleep/wake pattern. **307.44 Primary Hypersomnia** The predominant complaint is difficulty initiating or maintaining sleep or non-restorative sleep for at least 1 month, documented on polysomnogram (PSG) and multiple sleep latency test (MSLT), with short latencies but no REM abnormalities. **347 Narcolepsy** Falls asleep inappropriately, cataplexy, hypnagogic hallucinations, sleep paralysis, documented on PSG and MSLT, with short latency and sleep onset REM. **307.47 Dyssomnia, Not Otherwise Specified** (see *DSM-IV* Criteria Appendix, p 325)	**Infancy and Early Childhood** Rarely recognized at this age. **Middle Childhood and Adolescence** *Narcolepsy* may present at this age with a gradual, although rarely abrupt, onset of daytime sleepiness manifest by either: 1) the resumption of daytime naps that had been discontinued years previously without an obvious change in nighttime sleep quantity or quality, or 2) sleep inertia upon awakening. *Daytime cataplexy* may be present at the onset or soon after and may be described as "my legs feel like jello," most often associated with laughter. Hypnagogic hallucinations at sleep onset may be misdiagnosed as developing psychosis and are often very frightening, occasionally leading to sleep onset insomnia. Sleep onset paralysis is an uncommon complaint in children and adolescents. *Recurrent hypersomnia* (Kleine-Levin) may be preceded by a week or more of dysphoric and/or irritable behavior before the onset of hypersomnia. Episodes of hypersomnia tend to decrease in severity and frequency over time. *Delayed sleep phase* is more typically seen in adolescents who are often unable to fall asleep until 3 am. Once asleep, sleep appears normal, but the child is unable to awaken until 8 to 12 hours after sleep onset (11 am to 3 pm). Attempts by parents to awaken the adolescent are generally unsuccessful. The adolescent may be belligerent if forced to awaken. Social factors, work schedules, and refusal to attend school may play an important part in the maintenance of the disorder.

DIFFERENTIAL DIAGNOSIS	SPECIAL INFORMATION
General Medical Conditions Sleep is a highly regulated neurobehavioral process that can be disrupted by any factor that has a significant impact on the integrity or function of the central nervous system (CNS). Any CNS disease process that has an adverse impact on daytime waking function may also adversely affect nocturnal sleep and/or the ability to maintain wakefulness. Any condition that interferes with sleep onset, fragments nighttime sleep, interferes with the CNS, affects circadian phase, or increases sleep need may result in excessive daytime sleepiness. Examples include: Obstructive sleep apnea Encephalitis Meningitis Seizures Traumatic/metabolic brain injury Structural CNS disturbance Periodic movements of sleep Blindness Pain (acute or chronic) Infection	OSA/OHV causes excessive sleepiness during middle childhood and adolescence and is less common in younger children.
Substances Many medications may cause excessive sleepiness while they are being used. Examples include: Sedative hypnotics and anxiolytics (benzodiazepines, chloral hydrate) Tricyclic antidepressants (imipramine) Antihistamines (diphenhydramine) Anticonvulsants (phenobarbital) Alcohol Opioid Clonidine Some medications/drugs may cause temporary excessive sleepiness upon discontinuation. Methylphenidate Amphetamines Cocaine Some CNS toxins (e.g., lead) may cause excessive daytime sleepiness.	

DIFFERENTIAL DIAGNOSIS, CONTINUED	SPECIAL INFORMATION, CONTINUED
Mental Disorders Other mental disorders may include excessive sleepiness as one of their symptoms or complaints. Examples include: **296.xx** Major depressive disorder **296.xx** Bipolar I disorder, most recent episode depressed **307.44** Hypersomnia related to another mental disorder **307.47** Dyssomnia not otherwise specified **317, 318.x, 319** Mental retardation **347** Narcolepsy **307.44** Primary hypersomnia Delayed sleep phase syndrome **300.4** Mood disorders such as dysthymia	Many depressed adolescents complain of hypersomnia, but objective studies have generally failed to confirm this finding. Children with mental retardation often have significant disruptions in sleep/wake scheduling. In Prader Willi syndrome, excessive sleepiness is almost universal.

COMMONLY COMORBID CONDITIONS	SPECIAL INFORMATION
Other Comorbid Mental Health Conditions — Examples include: **313.81** Oppositional defiant disorder **312.81** Conduct disorder childhood onset **312.82** Conduct disorder adolescent onset **317, 318.xx, 319** Mental retardation **307.42** Primary insomnia **300.02** Generalized anxiety disorder **314.xx** Attention-deficit/hyperactivity disorder	A number of behavioral syndromes labeled as mental health problems or disorders occur in children with excessive sleepiness. The association may be secondary to an inadequate amount of total sleep.
Other General Medical Conditions Medical problems that contribute to obstructive sleep apnea/obstructive hyperventilation. Examples include: Midfacial hypoplasia Retroganthia Adenotonsillar hypertrophy Hypotonia Craniofacial anomalies Laryngotracheomalacia Obesity Pharyngeal flap repair of cleft palate Status after upper airway burn/trauma	

Presenting Complaints

Refusing/not wanting to go to sleep
Cannot (get to) sleep
Stalling or dawdling at bedtime
Disruptive/inconsistent attention to bedtime routine
Somatic complaints at bedtime ("stomachache," "headache,"
  "don't feel good")
"Not tired"
Nervous or worried
Frightened (of bad dreams)

Definition and Symptoms

Insomnia is the inability to fall asleep (sleep onset insomnia) at a reasonable and appropriate time for age or level of development and/or the inability to stay asleep (sleep maintenance) or to fall back asleep after awakening during the night. Symptoms may include stalling, repetitive getting up out of bed before falling asleep, calling for the parent, requesting food or water unnecessarily, complaints of aches or pains not present any other time of day, expressions of agitation including nervousness, fear of bad dreams, or more global fears that something will "happen" while asleep.

Delayed sleep phase syndrome is a circadian rhythm condition during which the major sleep time is delayed in relation to desired clock time, resulting in symptoms of sleep onset insomnia and/or difficulty in awakening in the morning.

Restless legs is a well-defined problem in adults which is often reported to have begun during childhood. It is described as an unpleasant dysesthesia generally involving the legs which is present at sleep onset and may interfere with the transition to sleep. It may be associated with periodic movements of sleep which are brief (0.5 to 5.0 seconds), periodic movements of the lower extremity which may be associated with arousals.

Partial arousal conditions include a spectrum of clinical phenomena that occur along a spectrum from quiet sleepwalking to sleep terrors. These disorders represent a sudden partial arousal usually at the end of a period of slow-wave sleep. Behaviorally, the child is unaware of and unresponsive to the environment. The duration of the arousal varies from 30 seconds to 20 minutes and generally terminates with the child's return to sleep without ever fully awakening. The child is generally amnestic for the arousal the following morning. There is often a positive family history for partial arousals.

Epidemiology and Etiology

Normally, children are excellent sleepers, falling asleep quickly, sleeping quietly and peacefully through the night without obvious behavioral arousals; and awake refreshed the following morning. However, what may appear as a uniform uninterrupted sleep period is actually comprised of a series of 60- to 90-minute cycles during which the child experiences both non-rapid eye movement (non-REM) and REM sleep. The proportions of REM and non-REM sleep vary across the night, with the majority of non-REM sleep occurring in the first one third of the night, and the majority of REM sleep occurring in the second half of the night. In most children, these cycles are seamlessly woven together to form the night's sleep. During the night it is normal for there to be 5 to 10 brief, behaviorally inapparent arousals in a child who "sleeps through" the night. However, the weave can be disrupted such that there is difficulty either at the transitions from wake to sleep, during the night, at the transition from one sleep stage to another, or after a brief arousal. Anxiety, depression, circadian factors, disorders of arousal, medical/neurologic problems, and drugs all may play a role in the disruption of normal sleep onset and sleep maintenance. These factors are often cumulative.

Most insomnia in infants, children, and adolescents is phenomenologically different from insomnia in adults as the problem is usually a result of interactional and perceptual difficulties between the caregiver and the child and/or the child and his or her environment.

DEVELOPMENTAL VARIATION	COMMON DEVELOPMENTAL PRESENTATIONS
V65.49 Insomnia/Sleeplessness Variation Insomnia—difficulty falling asleep or returning to sleep—is considered a developmental variation if the symptom is clearly different from the child's (previous) pattern of sleep, can usually be related to or associated with an obvious source or stimulus (such as an acute medical problem or identified stressor), is not having a significant or enduring impact on the child's daytime behavior or development, or adversely affecting the parents' sleep, and is self-limited.	**Infancy** Most infants and toddlers start to sleep through the night between 3 and 6 months of age. An increase of night waking is common in the second 6 months of the first year of life, and it is estimated that one fourth to one third of toddlers between 1 and 2 years of age still awaken during the night. Partial arousals are common at this age and present as sudden awakenings often associated with a considerable degree of agitation, walking and/or running, and talking or mumbling, usually in the first one third of the night. The child is often unable to be aroused and unresponsive during these partial arousals. The duration is typically brief (1 to 10 minutes), and the child will rapidly return to a quiet sleep. These symptoms may be very frightening to parents who often will try to force the child awake, which may escalate the agitated behavior. Common daily life stressors, including minor intercurrent illnesses as well as major life changes (starting school, divorce, death in the family, change of living environment or day care arrangements) may result in disruption of normal sleep patterns. **Early Childhood** Nightmares are common during preschool and early childhood years and are frequently associated with frightening events from a child's daily life or from having viewed frightening movies or television programs. Nightmares typically awaken children in the later part of the night at which time they are usually alert, frightened, and able to describe their dreams vividly. Recall of nightmares and anticipatory anxiety about a recurrent bad dream may interfere with the ability of the child to fall back to sleep easily or to initiate sleep at bedtime on subsequent nights. These usually are isolated occurences that become problematic if they become recurrent. **Middle Childhood** The challenges of normal development in school-age children increase the possibility of stress, worries, fears, and phobias as natural parts of their growth and development. Such anxieties may evolve easily into difficulty falling asleep, an appearance or increase in night-wakenings as seen with "nightmares," and associated difficulty in falling back asleep after awakening in the night. Such stressors also may contribute to an increase in existing parasomnias, i.e., disorders of arousal. Restless legs may first present during childhood or adolescence as nonspecific leg pains or leg cramps at bedtime when the child is lying in bed, or as "growing pains" during the day. This dysesthesia may interfere with sleep onset and cause the child to want to get up and walk around. **Adolescence** As with the other pediatric age groups, sleep disturbances may be related to symptoms of acute or chronic illness, stresses of life change events, or the effects of drugs, prescribed or illicit. In addition, difficulty with sleep may be an early sign of a major emotional disorder appearing at this time, such as anorexia nervosa, major depressive disorder, or schizophrenia. Insomnia during adolescence is often a function of anxiety from a variety of sources and reflective of the unique developmental challenges of adolescence. Irregular sleep/wake schedules and chronic sleep deprivation secondary to social, academic, and employment demands are the norm in American adolescents. These sources together with a physiologic

DEVELOPMENTAL VARIATION, CONTINUED	COMMON DEVELOPMENTAL PRESENTATIONS, CONTINUED
	delay in sleep phase put adolescents at a particular risk for developing sleep difficulties. Most adolescents adapt to these demands with sleep restriction during the school week and sleeping in on weekends, but some adolescents appear unable to alter their sleep onset and arousal times substantially over the course of a week. These teens develop severe sleep deprivation and are at particular risk for developing a delayed sleep phase syndrome.

SPECIAL INFORMATION

Beyond sleep association disorders, common medical conditions of infancy and young children (and their treatments) typically contribute to or cause both sleep onset insomnia and disruption of sleep in association with their other symptoms. Thus, any medical problem causing pain or discomfort (e.g., fever) may prevent or disrupt sleep. Prevalence varies with the relative prevalence of various medical problems. In infancy these most commonly include respiratory infections in which discomfort and difficulty with breathing may make falling asleep problematic, otitis media with effusion, gastroesophageal reflux, and colic, along with a myriad of other illnesses.

Infants who consistently fall asleep while being nursed, bottle fed, rocked, or held may experience delay in sleep onset because of these activities and/or may be unable to return to sleep after a normal arousal without the caregiver recreating the sleep onset association. Because 5 to 10 brief arousals during the night are normal for an infant, this may result in many awakenings during the night for both the child and caregiver.

In preschoolers limit-setting sleep requirements are the most common source of difficulty "falling asleep" or getting to sleep when sleep readiness is physiologically evident. These are often manifest in "stalling tactics," with requests for more hugs and kisses, drinks of water, or stories. While these problems typically quickly become habituated as a result of misunderstanding or inadequate/insufficient limit-setting by the caregiver, recent or new onset of the same behaviors must also be understood as possible manifestations of an anxiety/ stress/worry problem, and/or the result of an experienced or fantasized trauma of some kind. Life change events such as divorce, remarriage, the move to a new home, parental illness, financial/ work stressors, birth of a new baby, and death in the family are commonly disruptive of all routines, including sleep patterns. Sleep may also be affected by other major changes in the developmental life of a child, such as toilet training, starting school, returning to school after a vacation, or going to camp.

Parental beliefs, misconceptions, and unrealistic expectations play a prominent role in the understanding and inadvertent perpetuation of insomnia or sleeplessness in developmentally normal, healthy children. A sleep journal recording timing, duration, and associated parental and child behaviors and feelings at bedtime (and during night wakings) will facilitate both understanding and management of these common problems.

During adolescence circadian factors and sleep deprivation play an important role in sleep quality. A sleep log prospectively documenting the timing of sleep onset and sleep duration over a period of a couple of weeks will help in understanding the circadian influences on sleep.

DEVELOPMENTAL VARIATION, CONTINUED	SPECIAL INFORMATION, CONTINUED
	Travel across more than three time zones, especially eastward, is the most common cause of a transient circadian problem that may result in difficulties at sleep onset as well as frequent nocturnal arousals or excessive daytime sleepiness.
	Medical problems, and especially those that do not resolve as predicted or those known to be chronic, typically may delay or prevent sleep onset (or disrupt sleep maintenance), both by the discomfort associated with the problem (e.g., abdominal pain, diarrhea, difficulty swallowing, asthma) and by the attendant anxiety about the course or status of the illness. Chronic illnesses such as cystic fibrosis, diabetes mellitus, asthma, leukemia, or other cancers may affect sleep in children through several mechanisms, including direct effects of the illness on the central nervous system (CNS) regulation of sleep, effects of disruption of sleep schedules because of and during hospitalizations, and effects of anxiety and family interactional difficulties related to the child's illness.

PROBLEM	COMMON DEVELOPMENTAL PRESENTATIONS
V40.3 Insomnia/Sleeplessness Problem, Partial Arousals Problem Insomnia—difficulty falling asleep or returning to sleep—is considered a problem if the symptom begins to have an impact or adverse effect on the child's daytime behavior or development, or is so disruptive to the parents' sleep such that it has a negative effect upon their daytime behavior or functioning but is not of sufficient intensity to qualify for a diagnosis of primary insomnia or dysomnia, NOS. The latter tends to be more common than the former in infancy and early and middle childhood.	**Infancy** The majority of the problematic awakenings result from sleep onset association problems (in which the child inadvertently becomes reliant/dependent on the caregiver to help complete the transition from wakefulness to sleep). With the developmental task of achieving object permanence, separation anxiety may present between the ages of 10 to 24 months with the new onset of difficulty falling asleep at bedtime or of returning to sleep during the night in a child who previously had fallen asleep easily. When sleep onset is prolonged beyond their expectation of what is normal or "usual" (beyond 30 minutes), parental tension is heightened, evening "relaxation" may be delayed, disrupted, or prevented, and parental discord is increased. All of these stressors may in turn contribute to disruption of parental sleep patterns, parental resentment and confusion, and subsequent parent-child interactional difficulties. **Early and Middle Childhood** School-age children may reflect persistence of the limit-setting sleep disorders that have not been attended to. Insomnia that appears or persists into school-age years almost invariably is secondary to anxiety about other life changes or stressors, or to some other disorder. Parental understanding and acceptance of the stimulus and origin of the problem, and their personal effectiveness in coping usually allow for easier resolution of the child's problem. Partial arousals, if occurring frequently and/or associated with a severe agitation, can be very disruptive for the parent who can then inadvertently transmit these anxieties to the child who previously was likely to be unaware of the arousal. This reaction may be a perpetuating factor leading to maintenance of the arousals, and may contribute to anxiety at sleep onset. **Adolescence** Chronic sleep restriction, chaotic sleep/wake scheduling, and the development of a delayed sleep phase may commonly have an adverse impact on an adolescent's sleep continuity, may be self-perpetuating, and may result in severe sleep restriction that leads to excessive daytime sleepiness, which affects functioning in school, at work, and in social relationships.

PROBLEM, CONTINUED	SPECIAL INFORMATION
	The tensions and worries of middle childhood may both exacerbate existing or unresolved sleeplessness and cause insomnia as a reflection of those anxieties. Children between ages 8 and 11 years may have insomnia in association with a form of separation anxiety related to their emerging understanding and conceptualization of the finality and permanency of death. Thus, both real and symbolic losses (e.g., divorce, family moves, new house, loss of friends, death of a relative or friend, loss of ideal) may have a profound symptomatic impact different from earlier childhood experiences.
	Parents who are awakened several times a night to reestablish their infant's sleep onset association often suffer from sleep fragmentation and sleep deprivation, while their infants and toddlers do not typically suffer any ill effects from these frequent night wakenings. Parents may differ considerably (from one another) in their view of the problem and their willingness to participate in the solution through modification of their own beliefs and behaviors.
	In all age groups there is a risk that acute situational insomnia (e.g., as due to family/environmental change, illness, side effect of medication) that either goes unrecognized or mismanaged may easily become conditioned, resulting in a chronic insomnia problem. Early diagnosis and prompt, appropriate management should prevent such conditioning from developing into a chronic insomnia.
	Persistence of a limit-setting sleep problem that has not been attended to may be seen in children who consistently request, demand, and succeed in sleeping in their parents' bed at night. This behavior ordinarily reflects a conditioned response based on difficulties in parental limit-setting, and may be perpetuated/exacerbated by parental anxieties/needs, and/or by everyday tensions in the child's or family's life.
	If infants, toddlers, and preschoolers are put to bed and expected to sleep longer than their nocturnal sleep requirement, they may experience "insomnia" with delays in sleep onset, have difficulty returning to sleep after awakening in the night, or awaken early in the morning.

DISORDER	COMMON DEVELOPMENTAL PRESENTATIONS
307.42 Primary Insomnia • The predominant complaint is difficulty initiating or maintaining sleep for at least 1 month. • The sleep disturbance causes clinically significant distress or impairment in functioning. • The sleep disturbance does not occur exclusively during the course of narcolepsy, breathing-related sleep disorder, circadian rhythm sleep disorder, or a parasomnia. • The disturbance does not occur exclusively during the course of another mental disorder (e.g., major depressive disorder, generalized anxiety disorder, or delirium). **307.47 Dyssomnia, Not Otherwise Specified** Insomnia that does not meet criteria for any specific dyssomnia, including: • Complaints of clinically significant insomnia attributable to environmental factors, e.g., noise, light, frequent interruptions (as in chaotic households). • Excess sleepiness attributable to ongoing sleep deprivation. • Idiopathic "restless legs syndrome": uncomfortable sensations that lead to an intense urge to move the legs, typically beginning before sleep onset, relieved with walking; can delay sleep or awaken the child from sleep. • Situations in which the clinician has concluded that a dyssomnia is present but is unable to determine whether it is primary, due to a general medical condition, or substance induced. **307.45 Circadian Rhythm Sleep Disorder (Formerly Sleep-Wake Schedule Disorder)** (see *DSM-IV* Criteria, Appendix, p 325)	**Infancy** Infants with *circadian rhythm sleep disorder* fall asleep early in the evening (not usually either noticed or considered a problem by parents), awaken early in the morning, and also have naptime and mealtime problems in that they are shifted to an earlier time. This advanced sleep phase problem occurs mainly in infants and toddlers and is quite common. *Primary insomnia* and *dyssomnia* in infancy are almost unheard of and represent diagnoses of exclusion. **Early Childhood** In *dyssomnia, NOS,* younger children in chaotic households may have frequent night awakenings and/or vague reports of nightmares associated with the anxiety and uncertainty of frequent and inconsistent adult comings and goings in the home. For *circadian rhythm sleep disorder,* young children may manifest difficulty going to sleep at night and trouble awakening "on time" for daycare or preschool in the morning. Parents may learn from day care providers that such children nap earlier and/or longer than other children. **Middle Childhood** Older children with delayed sleep phase circadian rhythm disorders may complain of insomnia but also have considerable difficulty awakening in the morning. In addition to major arguments and "battles" around waking up in time for school, daytime sleepiness in school may be a presenting problem and clue to diagnosis. Children with circadian rhythm disorders may go to bed cooperatively and be unable to fall asleep for a long time. Unlike the similar behavior in a limit-setting sleep disorder, this particular manifestation is absent in circadian rhythm disorders when bedtime is sufficiently late. Children with this disorder also may seem to get a "second wind" right before bedtime, then fight or "stall," and not be able to fall asleep because they are wide awake. **Adolescence** Morning wake-up difficulties and difficulties staying awake during school are especially typical of and dramatic in teenagers with circadian rhythm disorders. The adolescent with rare idiopathic insomnia may reflect poor concentration, impaired vigilance and attention, low energy, increased fatigue, and bad mood.
	SPECIAL INFORMATION
	Circadian rhythm sleep disorders include the uncommon occurrence of advanced sleep phase problem, mainly noted in infants and toddlers and manifest in falling asleep early (in the evening) and awakening very early in the morning. It is managed best by shifting (delaying) the timing of naps, mealtimes, and bedtime, and by light control. While most children with insomnia/sleeplessness have normal CNS function, some may have poor sleep in association with and as a result of severe CNS dysfunction as may be seen with cerebral injury, severe metabolic disorder, or congenital malformations. A variety of problems have associated sleep difficulties. Many totally blind individuals have a free-running circadian rhythm resulting in extreme difficulty or an inability to establish a regular sleep/wake schedule. Children with mental retardation, Prader-Willi syndrome, and Rett syndrome may have insomnia and night-waking. Delayed sleep phase syndrome can be a common cause of insomnia or delayed sleep onset in all age groups. Typically, in addition to

DISORDER, CONTINUED	SPECIAL INFORMATION, CONTINUED
	not falling asleep until late (and regularly so), older children and teenagers with this problem experience arguments and battles about waking up in time for school and daytime sleepiness.

DIFFERENTIAL DIAGNOSIS	SPECIAL INFORMATION
General Medical Conditions Sleep is a highly regulated neurobehavioral CNS process, easily disrupted by any factor significantly interfering with the integrity or function of the CNS. Examples include: Otitis media with effusion Respiratory illness (including upper respiratory infection, bronchiolitis, asthma, pneumonia, cystic fibrosis) Gastroesophageal reflux Colic Illnesses with associated discomfort, fever Obstructive sleep apnea Any condition that has an impact on the integrity of the CNS Neuromuscular diseases Chronic illness	Code Sleep Disorder — Insomnia due to a general medical condition **780.52.** True food allergy insomnia is an unusual disorder causing sleep disruption in the first few months of life, and is cured with the elimination of cow's milk. The sleep of preschoolers also may be influenced by many different medical problems, especially when fever or discomfort are prominent symptoms. Conditions causing respiratory difficulty sufficient to disrupt sleep include tonsillar (and adenoidal) enlargement, maxillofacial abnormalities, or obesity.
Substances Many medications may cause disruption of sleep, either as a side effect, effects of discontinuation/withdrawal of medication, or as paradoxical effects. Commonly used medications that may contribute to sleeplessness (falling asleep or returning to sleep) include: Caffeine in food or drugs (colas, other soft drinks, cocoa, coffee, tea) Asthma medications including theophylline products, ß2-agonists such as albuterol Sympathomimetics commonly found in cold and cough preparations (e.g., pseudoephedrine, phenylpropanolamine, etc.) Stimulants as commonly used for attentional disorders: methylphenidate, pemoline, dextroamphetamine Alcohol Propranolol Cocaine Discontinuation of/withdrawal from sedative hypnotics, benzodiazepines, chloral hydrate, alcohol Paradoxical effects of medications typically thought of and used as sedating may cause excitability and agitation leading to sleep onset insomnia and difficulty returning to sleep. Examples include barbiturates such as phenobarbital and antihistamines such as diphenhydramine.	In any age group, medications may contribute to restlessness or related symptoms. In school-age children and adolescents the use of stimulant medications for attention disorders (e.g., methylphenidate [if taken close to bedtime], pemoline, dextroamphetamine) may also contribute to sleeplessness. For most children these are transient side effects associated with acclimation to medication, but for some the sleeplessness may be sufficient to require either alteration of dosage or dosage schedules or change in medication.

DIFFERENTIAL DIAGNOSIS, CONTINUED	SPECIAL INFORMATION, CONTINUED
Mental Disorders Many additional mental disorders may include insomnia as one of their symptoms. Examples include: 308.30 Acute stress disorder 314.xx Attention-deficit/hyperactivity disorder 307.23 Tourette's disorder 780.59 Breathing-related sleep disorder 995.54 Physical abuse of child 995.53 Sexual abuse of child 995.52 Neglect of child 300.01 Panic disorder 296.2x Major depressive disorder — single episode 296.3x Major depressive disorder — recurrent 300.4 Dysthymic disorder 309.21 Separation anxiety disorder 300.02 Generalized anxiety disorder 300.0 Anxiety disorder, not otherwise specified 309.81 Posttraumatic stress disorder 309.xx Adjustment disorder	

COMMONLY COMORBID CONDITIONS	SPECIAL INFORMATION
Other Comorbid Mental Health Conditions	Since insomnia is a common symptom of some other mental disorders, it usually is not considered as a separate diagnosis if the mental disorder is present. In most cases code the mental disorder only.
Other General Medical Conditions — Examples include: Pain Chronic illness/infection Blindness Mental retardation	

Presenting Complaints

awakening from sleep

sleepwalking

sleep terrors

sleep apnea

nightmares

head banging/body rocking

inability to fall asleep

nocturnal eating/drinking

Definitions and Symptoms

Nocturnal arousals are best understood within the context of the normal sleep cycle. This cycle is about 60 minutes long in infants and increases to 90 minutes during adolescence. Within each cycle the child will have both non-rapid eye movement non-(REM)/dream sleep and REM sleep. Non-REM sleep can be further subdivided into stages I and IV, roughly paralleling the depth of sleep. Non-REM stages III and IV are together described as slow-wave sleep. Although the periodicity of non-REM/REM cycles remains regular throughout the night, the amount of time spent in each and the distribution of non-REM, stage I, stage II, stage III, and stage IV changes over the night. After each non-REM to REM sleep cycle, it is not unusual for there to be a brief, although behaviorally inapparent, arousal. Thus the nighttime sleep, although it appears continuous, is made up of a series of 5 to 10 non-REM/REM cycles that are seamlessly woven together. Slow-wave sleep (non-REM stages III/IV sleep) predominates in the first third of the night, and REM (dream) sleep predominates in the latter third.

Brief arousals for feeding are a normal part of an infant's sleep cycle, and brief, behaviorally inapparent arousals are a normal part of everyone's sleep cycle. Arousals become a clinical problem when either a child is unable to return to sleep after a normal arousal or the arousal is caused by an underlying medical, neurological, or psychiatric problem.

Slow-Wave Sleep (non-REM stage III and IV sleep)

Slow-wave sleep is defined polygraphically when the EEG is synchronized with high voltage (>50 uv) slow waves (0.5.2 Hz). Behaviorally it appears as quiet sleep with regular respiration and heart rate and very little spontaneous movement. Slow-wave sleep duration and depth vary with age, predominating in both intensity and duration during infancy and diminishing to adult levels by the end of adolescence.

Partial Arousal Disorders

Partial arousal disorders include a spectrum of clinical phenomena that occur along a spectrum from quiet sleepwalking to night terrors. These disorders represent a sudden partial arousal usually at the end of a period of slow-wave sleep. Behaviorally, the child is unaware of and unresponsive to the environment. The duration of the arousal varies from 30 seconds to 20 minutes and generally terminates with the child returning to sleep without ever fully awakening. The child is generally amnestic for the arousal the following morning. There is often a family history of partial arousals.

Head banging and body rocking are rhythmic movements that generally occur at sleep onset and after normal nocturnal arousals during the night, although they may be present during sleep. The movements may be accompanied by moaning, which can be particularly disruptive to caregivers. These movements are common during infancy, but the prevalence decreases with age.

DEVELOPMENTAL VARIATION	COMMON DEVELOPMENTAL PRESENTATIONS

V65.49 Nocturnal Arousals Variation

Nocturnal arousals are considered a developmental variation if a child is consistently arousing from sleep after 9 months of age, and if the arousals are self-limited, brief, usually associated with an obvious acute medical problem, and are not having a significant impact on the child's daytime behavior, development, daytime sleep, or adversely affecting the parents' sleep.

Infancy

Infants learn to fall asleep and often develop onset associations with certain activities such as feeding, rocking, sucking on a pacifier, etc. It is normal for nocturnal arousals to occur in infants after each sleep cycle. Partial arousals may be evident as brief periods of unexplained crying during the first third of the night, during which time the infant appears unresponsive to the parent and will not return to sleep easily.

Early and Middle Childhood

Once the child is out of the crib, he or she is able to seek out the parents during the night. This is a behavior that can be easily and quickly conditioned by inadvertent reinforcement such as allowing the child to sleep with the parents. If the total time in bed is longer than the total requisite sleep time, there may be long periods during the night the child is awake. Some children may get out of bed and play or watch television. If the children are quiet or do not complain, the parents may be unaware of the awakenings.

Adolescence

Partial arousals may be triggered by irregular sleep-wake schedule, sleep deprivation, or stress, all of which are common during adolescence. These arousals may be more violent than at younger ages. The peak prevalence in quiet sleepwalking is in early adolescence. Sleep onset association may include listening to music or watching television and may result in an inability to consolidate sleep.

SPECIAL INFORMATION

Excessive nighttime feeding (> 8 oz) may result in conditioned hunger and excessive wetting in addition to problems with sleep onset associations. Infantile colic is a common problem affecting up to 50% of infants between the ages of 2 weeks and 3 months of age. In the majority of these children, the crying occurs in the evening and resolves by bedtime; however, 12% of infants with colic will have episodes beginning at night and 8% will have episodes occurring randomly throughout the day and night. Separation anxiety may present after age 9 months with the new onset of nocturnal arousals in a child who previously slept well throughout the night. Although most infants are physiologically capable of consolidating 6 to 10 hours of sleep at night, 30% are still waking at least nightly by 1 year of age. Sixty percent of children have exhibited some rhythmic movements at sleep onset or during the night by 9 months of age. This decreases over time, and by 2 years of age, 22% are engaged in some regular, rhythmic movements during the night. If infants are put in bed and expected to sleep longer than their nocturnal sleep need, they may experience delays with sleep onset, have long periods of wakefulness during the night, or have an early morning awakening.

Circadian factors and sleep deprivation often plan an important role in sleep quality, especially during adolescence. A sleep log prospectively documenting the timing of sleep onset, frequency, and duration of nocturnal arousals and sleep duration kept over a period of 2 weeks or more is often invaluable in understanding the circadian influences on sleep.

DEVELOPMENTAL VARIATION, CONTINUED	SPECIAL INFORMATION, CONTINUED
	Nightmares become increasingly common at this age and are often associated with watching frightening television or movies. The child typically awakens in the later part of the night frightened but alert with a vivid recall of frightening imagery. Traveling across more than three time zones, especially in an eastward direction, is the most common cause of a transient circadian problem that may result in difficulties at sleep onset, frequent nocturnal arousals, or excessive daytime sleepiness.

PROBLEM	COMMON DEVELOPMENTAL PRESENTATIONS
V40.3 Nocturnal Arousals Problem Nocturnal arousals are a problem when they have an adverse impact on the child's daytime behavior and/or sleep, or are disruptive to the parents' sleep so that they begin to have an adverse impact on the parents' daytime behavior or functioning but are not sufficiently intense to qualify for the diagnosis of one of the nocturnal arousal disorders. The latter is more common than the former in infancy and early and middle childhood.	**Infancy** Parents who are awakened two or more times a night to reestablish their infant's sleep onset association often suffer from sleep deprivation and sleep fragmentation. Typically, their infants do not suffer any ill effects from these frequent arousals. Parents often differ substantially in their view of the problems and their willingness to participate in the solution. Infants taking more than 16 ounces of formula per night often develop conditioned hunger during the night and become excessively wet, causing discomfort and arousal. Some children are unable to return to sleep after this normal arousal unless their sleep onset associations are reestablished. If the sleep onset association involves the parent and the infant is unable to return to sleep on his or her own, the result is the infant crying until the parent reestablishes the sleep onset association. Once the sleep onset associations are reestablished, the infant will rapidly return to sleep. This may recur throughout the night after each spontaneous awakening. **Early and Middle Childhood** Partial arousals may appear more frequent and/or be associated with more autonomic arousals during early and middle childhood. The child may have had other manifestations of partial arousals at a younger age. The greatest risk to the child is potential injury. Children who are consistently sleeping in their parents' bed at night at this age may be responding to the parents' needs. Head banging and body rocking rarely represent serious pathology, although they may disrupt the sleep of other family members. **Adolescence** The combined effect of chronic sleep restriction, chaotic sleep/wake scheduling, and the development of a delayed sleep phase, all of which are common during adolescence, can have an adverse impact on an adolescent's sleep continuity resulting in frequent arousals and can affect their daytime behavior. Partial arousals may become increasingly violent and may lead to substantial injuries or endangering behavior.

SPECIAL INFORMATION
When separation anxiety is severe, the parent may need to sleep in the child's room at least temporarily while the problem is being addressed. Head banging/body rocking may be frequent and/or

PROBLEM, CONTINUED	SPECIAL INFORMATION, CONTINUED
	violent in a small number of children but is rarely associated with significant injury in neurologically normal children and is rarely due to psychological or psychiatric disorders.
	Parents who are unable to set reasonable limits for their children during the day will often have the same problem with limit setting at night — both at sleep onset and after an arousal. Partial arousals are often more dramatic during early and middle childhood than in infancy. The behavior may vary from quiet sleepwalking to agitated sleep terrors. Triggers may include sleep deprivation, disrupted sleep schedule, or acute illness. The primary concern is safety, and the parent needs to ensure the child is not in danger. Head banging and body rocking decrease to 5% by 5 years of age. Restless legs and periodic movements of sleep may first become apparent during early and middle childhood. At this age, the child is first able to describe the dysesthesias of restless legs syndrome. The description may be of nonspecific leg pains, growing pains, or an inability to keep legs still at sleep onset or when sedentary during the day. Generally, the child is unaware of the periodic leg movements during the night, although the parents might be aware of them if they have slept with their child or observed the child closely during sleep.
	Physical and/or sexual abuse (see p 45) may result in dissociative states that manifest as unusual nocturnal arousals. The sleep environment is an important part of the assessment of sleep problems. The presence of television, radio, telephone, and the amount of natural light the child receives may all be important factors.

DISORDER	COMMON DEVELOPMENTAL PRESENTATIONS
307.46 Sleep Terror Disorder Recurrent episodes of abrupt awakening from sleep, usually occurring during the first third of the major sleep episodes and beginning with a panicky scream. • Intense fear and signs of autonomic arousal such as tachycardia, rapid breathing, and sweating. • Relative unresponsiveness to efforts to comfort. • No detailed dream recall and amnesia for the episode. • Episodes cause clinically significant distress or impairment. **307.46 Sleepwalking Disorder** Repeated episodes of rising from bed during sleep and walking about, usually occurring in the first third of the major sleep period. • While sleepwalking, the person has a blank staring face, is relatively unresponsive to the efforts of others, and can be awakened only with great difficulty. • On awakening, the person has amnesia for the episode. • The sleepwalking causes clinically significant distress or impairment. **307.47 Parasomnia, Not Otherwise Specified** REM sleep behavior disorder (RBD): motor activity, often violent in nature, that arises during REM sleep. Unlike sleepwalking, these episodes tend to occur later in the night and are associated with vivid dream recall.	**Infancy** These disorders are rarely described during infancy. **Early Childhood** Sleepwalking and sleep terrors may put a child in harm's way (leaving the house in winter, running into a window, etc.), which may be extremely upsetting to parents who are unable to "help" the child during an event. **Middle Childhood and Adolescence** Sleepwalking and sleep terrors may be quite common, up to several episodes per night. Injuries may result from violent episodes. These episodes usually have very little impact on the child's waking behavior. Posttraumatic stress disorder will often have sleep-related symptoms in children — either fears at sleep onset or recurrent nightmares that may disrupt and restrict sleep enough to cause secondary daytime sleepiness. Parents of children with attention-deficit disorders often complain of a variety of sleep problems including difficulties with sleep onset and frequent nocturnal arousals. Children with Tourette's disorder have a higher incidence of sleepwalking and sleep terrors. Tics often occur during sleep. Irregular sleep-wake schedules and sleep deprivation are the norm during adolescence, which may exacerbate the sleep terror and sleepwalking. **SPECIAL INFORMATION** Utilize the parasomnia, NOS code if the sleep behaviors are of sufficient intensity to warrant a disorder diagnosis but the behaviors are not characterized by sleepwalking or night terrors and if it is not possible to determine whether the symptoms are due to a medical illness or a substance.

DIFFERENTIAL DIAGNOSIS	SPECIAL INFORMATION
General Medical Conditions Sleep is a highly regulated neurobehavioral central nervous system process that can be disrupted by any factor that has a significant impact on the integrity or function of the central nervous system. Any disease process (structural, toxic, metabolic, infectious, or traumatic) that has an adverse impact on daytime waking function may also have an adverse impact on nocturnal sleep and/or the ability to maintain wakefulness. Any condition that fragments nighttime sleep may result in frequent nocturnal arousals. Examples include: Acute/serous otitis media Seizures Obstructive sleep apnea Asthma Milk allergy Periodic movement of sleep Neuromuscular disease Gastroesophageal reflux	In young children, either acute or serous otitis media is the most common medical condition that causes acute sleep fragmentation. Gastroesophageal reflux in infants and young children is another common cause of sleep fragmentation. Seizures may be exclusively nocturnal and may present with repetitive, stereotypical nocturnal arousals and/or behaviors that must be differentiated from sleep terrors. Other medical problems include acute infectious illness, obstructive sleep apnea, asthma, or periodic movements of sleep. Neuromuscular diseases, such as muscular dystrophy, may cause nocturnal hypoventilation that results in nocturnal arousals. Milk allergy in infants may cause short nighttime sleep and frequent nocturnal arousals alone or in addition to eczema, wheezing, vomiting, and diarrhea. These problems respond dramatically to a milk-free and often soy-free diet.
Substances Many medications may cause sleep fragmentation. Examples include: Stimulants (methylphenidate, pemoline, dexedrine) Asthma medications (theophylline, ß-blockers) Alcohol Caffeine Propranolol Cocaine Discontinuation of some medications (sedative hypnotics, benzodiazepines, chloral hydrate and alcohol) may result in sleep fragmentation	Paradoxical effects of medication, normally thought of as sedating, such as phenobarbital and antihistamines, may cause nocturnal arousals.
Mental Disorders Many other mental disorders include nocturnal arousals as one of their symptoms or associated features. Examples include: **309.81** Posttraumatic stress disorder **308.3** Acute stress disorder **300.02** Generalized anxiety disorder **299.00** Autism **307.45** Circadian rhythm disorder, delayed sleep phase type **307.47** Nighttime disorder **314.xx** Attention-deficit/hyperactivity disorder	

COMMONLY COMORBID CONDITIONS	SPECIAL INFORMATION
Other Comorbid Mental Health Conditions	Since it is common to have nocturnal arousals as part of other mental disorders, it will be uncommon to have it occur simultaneously with other mental disorders. In most cases, code the other mental disorder only.
Other General Medical Conditions Medical problems that may predispose a child to obstructive sleep apnea may be associated with nocturnal arousals, including enlarged tonsils and adenoids, midfacial hypoplasia, retroganthia, hypotonia/hypertonia, craniofacial anomalies, and obesity.	

Feeding, Eating, Elimination Behaviors

Soiling Problems

Day/Nighttime Wetting Problems

Purging/Binge Eating

Dieting/Body Image Problems

Irregular Feeding Behaviors

SOILING PROBLEMS

Presenting Complaints

soiling problems
constipation
stool passed other than in the toilet
soiling clothes
soiling bed

Definitions and Symptoms

Although in the majority of instances encopresis is associated with constipation, it occasionally occurs in its absence. Parents often do not recognize the underlying problem of constipation, and it is essential that the problem is clarified during evaluation of a child with soiling problems. Often a history of constipation has existed for a year or more before soiling begins. For 50% of children with encopresis, constipation occurs during the toddler years. There is also often a family history of constipation or other intestinal motility problems. Children with severe encopresis may have an abnormal and prolonged external anal sphincter contraction while straining to defecate (animus), which may lead to ineffective rectal evacuation and, therefore, fecal accumulation. Chronic fecal accumulation leads to dilatation and eventual incompetence of the internal sphincter, which is responsible for involuntary control of stool passage. This leaves only the external sphincter, which requires voluntary control (conscious effort) to prevent soiling. Children may be able to exert some voluntary control in the presence of peer pressure, but this is at the expense of directed attention to learning. Therefore, parents may complain that children only soil at home and not in school. Some families note the onset of constipation when a toddler switches from breast milk to cow's milk formula. Certain "constipating" foods may cause more problems for children with intrinsically slow intestinal motility than for those with normal motility. Such motility problems may be related to abnormalities of regulatory gastrointestinal peptides. With respect to developmental considerations, the passage of feces into inappropriate places may occur in the course of usual toilet training or in the presence of mental disorders such as mental retardation. There are two types of encopresis included in *DSM-IV:* **787.6** encopresis with constipation and overflow incontinence, and **307.7** encopresis without constipation and overflow incontinence. The second type is more likely to be associated with psychological factors, such as the presence of oppositional defiant disorder, and to be intentional rather than involuntary. A camping trip may trigger avoidance of stooling in young children unfamiliar with or afraid of outdoor toilets.

Because of its unpleasant nature, soiling is likely to be associated with other behavior problems and family disagreements. A child who has been previously toilet trained and begins soiling is likely to hide soiled garments or deny having soiled them. The longer soiling continues, the longer the time required for treatment. Careful attention to disimpaction, maintenance of clean-out, prescribed toileting, and diet is necessary for at least a year in the average patient. If there is a family history of constipation, the child and family may need to be counseled regarding life-time management.

Differential Diagnosis and Common Associated Conditions

Enuresis is often associated with encopresis. This may be more severe in children who have large amounts of retained feces. It is important to rule out the presence of medical conditions such as diastematomyelia, anterior placement of the anus, neurofibromatosis, lead poisoning, and hypothyroidism before embarking on the treatment of soiling and constipation. Certain medications such as iron, ritalin, imipramine, neuroleptics, or other anticholinergic drugs may trigger or exacerbate constipation.

Epidemiology

Approximately 1% of 5-year-olds have encopresis. The disorder is more common in males than in females.

DEVELOPMENTAL VARIATION	COMMON DEVELOPMENTAL PRESENTATIONS
V65.49 Soiling Variation The occasional passage of a small amount of feces inappropriately such that it soils the child's clothing or bedding. This situation usually will be associated with some circumstance such as not having access to toilet facilities.	**Infancy** Not relevant at this age. **Early Childhood** Toilet training for bowel movements usually begins around 2 years of age but wide variation up to 4 years of age can occur. The child passes stool in places other than in the toilet. **Middle Childhood** Occasional accidents can occur when children are preoccupied with other activities and do not have immediate access to toilet facilities. **Adolescence** Accidents in soiling are not likely to happen in normal situations unless there is a gastrointestinal illness such as diarrhea.
	SPECIAL INFORMATION
	Constipation may develop in transition between formula and cow's milk. Acute diarrheal illness may be associated with a soiling accident.

PROBLEM	COMMON DEVELOPMENTAL PRESENTATIONS
V40.3 Soiling Problem This symptom is a problem if it increases in frequency or causes disruption in parent-child or peer interactions but is not sufficiently intense to qualify for the diagnosis of encopresis.	**Infancy** Not relevant at this age. **Early Childhood** The child frequently has constipation, with or without soiling, and begins to fear or is preoccupied with toileting. **Middle Childhood** The child frequently has constipation, with or without soiling, and begins to fear or is preoccupied with toileting, has irregular stools, and has accidents; parents are concerned. **Adolescence** The adolescent frequently has constipation, with or without soiling, and begins to fear or be preoccupied with toileting.
	SPECIAL INFORMATION
	Chronic constipation may result from an inappropriate diet. Mild "soiling" may be related only to poor hygiene. Punitive or humiliating efforts by parents to correct soiling may contribute to the problem. Stool may be withheld in new or uncomfortable toileting situation (e.g., camping or at school). Stool may also be held during play. Consider soiling problems secondary to environmental context, such as transient regressive behavior, acute stress, abuse, and neglect.

DISORDER	COMMON DEVELOPMENTAL PRESENTATIONS
307.7 Encopresis Without Constipation and Overflow Incontinence **787.6 Encopresis With Constipation and Overflow Incontinence** Repeated passage of feces into inappropriate places (e.g., clothing or floor) whether involuntary or intentional. At least one such event a month for at least 3 months. Chronological age is at least 4 years (or equivalent developmental level). Only diagnose encopresis when the behavior is not due exclusively to the direct physiological effects of a substance (e.g., laxatives) or a general medical condition except through a mechanism involving constipation.	**Infancy** Not relevant at this age. **Early Childhood** The child experiences soiling — with or without constipation. **Middle Childhood** The child experiences constipation and soiling, avoiding potential situations that may lead to embarrassment. The child may deny having accidents. **Adolescence** The adolescent experiences constipation and soiling and may be more subtle in how symptoms are hidden.

	SPECIAL INFORMATION
	The child must be at least 4 years old. Soiling without constipation is rare and is more common in males than in females. Inadequate, inconsistent toilet training and psychosocial stress may be predisposing factors. Voluntary soiling is usually associated with oppositional defiant disorder or conduct disorder (see Aggressive/Oppositional Behaviors cluster, p 119).

DIFFERENTIAL DIAGNOSIS	SPECIAL INFORMATION
General Medical Conditions — Examples include: Hirschsprung disease Dysmotility problems Diastematomyelia Spina bifida Previous anorectal surgery Cerebral palsy Seizure disorders Amyotonia congenita Anterior placement of the anus Fissure and other anal pathology Neurofibromatosis Hypothyroidism	Hirschsprung disease is almost always diagnosed by 5 years of age. Previous, healed surgery problems may persist as a learned avoidance of moving bowels.
Substances — Examples include: Anticholinergic side effects Iron Neuroleptics	Substances listed cause constipation that may result in accidental soiling.
Mental Disorders — Examples include: 317, Mental retardation 318.x, 319 299.00 Autistic disorder	

COMMONLY COMORBID CONDITIONS	SPECIAL INFORMATION
Other Comorbid Mental Health Conditions — Examples include: 307.6 Enuresis 312.81 Conduct disorder childhood onset 312.82 Conduct disorder adolescent onset 313.81 Oppositional defiant disorder 315.00 Reading disorder 315.1 Mathematics disorder 315.2 Disorder of written expression	Enuresis may be secondary to encopresis, but encopresis is not common with enuresis.
Other General Medical Conditions Not relevant.	If there is a medical condition, it is likely to have a causal relationship with the symptoms; therefore there will rarely be a comorbid medical condition.

Presenting Complaints

wets the bed

wets during the daytime

wets both day and night

wets pants

wets pants and bed

Definitions and Symptoms

Enuresis is the repeated involuntary or intentional voiding of urine into a bed or clothes. Nocturnal enuresis can be primary or secondary. A child with primary enuresis has never had consistently dry beds. A child with secondary or onset enuresis has nighttime wetting after a minimal 6-month period of dryness. This type is less common than primary enuresis and more likely to have a general medical explanation. Daytime wetting has been described as "dysfunctional voiding" or "uninhibited neurogenic bladder"; some children have been called "daytime dribblers."

A child who experiences repeated daytime wetting needs to be differentiated from the child who has an occasional accident related to some event. The major factor in daytime wetting is "holding on" behavior. These children may void only two to three times daily compared to the normal five to seven times. They often void incompletely, which may predispose them to bladder infection. Because daytime wetting is more obvious to peers, these children may be socially rejected and demonstrate more emotional problems. In girls, daytime wetting may be caused by improper voiding with pooling of urine into the vagina, and later leakage.

In the case of primary enuresis, 15% of children who wet will spontaneously achieve control over their enuresis each year. It is likely that the majority of cases of primary nocturnal enuresis are related to poorly understood neurodevelopmental or learning factors. Family history is frequently positive for nocturnal enuresis, particularly with father-son transmission. Because of the high frequency of primary bedwetting in preschoolers, it should be regarded as a normal developmental variation.

Epidemiology

The prevalence of enuresis at age 5 years is 7% for males and 3% for females; at age 10 years the prevalence is 3% for males and 2% for females. At age 18 years, the prevalence is 1% for males and less among females.

Etiology

The cause of delayed nocturnal bladder control has been attributed to small bladder capacity, antidiuretic hormone nocturnal deficiency, evening polydipsia, or not awakening. Chronic constipation is often associated with nocturnal enuresis. Sometimes large amounts of caffeinated beverages are ingested by children in the evening, and this is not recognized by parents as a contributing factor in nocturnal enuresis. Occasionally, children with nocturnal enuresis are found to have urinary tract infections, diabetes, anatomic defects in the urinary tract, seizures, or sleep apnea. In a child with secondary enuresis, particular attention should be paid to the presence of unrecognized constipation, hyperthyroidism, urinary tract infection, or sexual abuse as causes (see Environmental Situations Defined, p 31).

DEVELOPMENTAL VARIATION	COMMON DEVELOPMENTAL PRESENTATIONS
V65.49 Day or Nighttime Wetting Variation **Primary nocturnal enuresis** Enuresis is a normal developmental variation until early school years. Daytime wetting may reflect a child's preoccupation with play, "forgetting" to go to the toilet, or fear of the toilet. Bladder capacity increases as a child gets older. Secondary transient wetting may stem from minor stress or temporary behavioral regression and is associated with birth of a sibling.	**Infancy** Spontaneous voiding is normal in infancy. **Early Childhood** Daytime and nighttime wetting are common. **Middle Childhood** Nighttime wetting is infrequent and may need further evaluation. **Adolescence** Wetting during adolescence warrants evaluation.
	SPECIAL INFORMATION
	At nighttime, 25% of 5-year-olds still have wetting problems; 3% still have problems by age 12 years. High caffeine intake by preschoolers may contribute to wetting.

PROBLEM	COMMON DEVELOPMENTAL PRESENTATIONS
V40.3 Wetting Problem Wetting is a problem if a child is beginning to be teased by peers or starting to avoid social encounters, or the wetting causes parent-child interactional problems but the symptoms are not sufficiently intense to qualify for the diagnosis of enuresis.	**Infancy** Wetting should not be a problem. Parents may have inappropriate expectations about toilet training. **Early Childhood** The child has difficulty during or is resistant to toilet training, resulting in difficulties in parent-child interactions. **Middle Childhood** Day and/or nighttime wetting; parental concern. **Adolescence** Day and/or night wetting; parent and adolescent concern.
	SPECIAL INFORMATION
	Parent-child conflict over the management of the wetting can damage relationships and entrench the incontinence (see other family relationship problem, p 45). Wetting secondary to environmental factors may be associated with fears, transient regression with stress, abuse, neglect, or post-traumatic stress disorder (see Anxious Symptoms cluster, p 145). Secondary wetting is most frequent in younger children.

DISORDER	COMMON DEVELOPMENTAL PRESENTATIONS
307.6 Enuresis Repeated voiding of urine into bed or clothes (whether involuntary or intentional). The behavior is clinically significant as manifested by either a frequency of twice a week for at least three consecutive months or the presence of clinically significant distress or impairment in social, academic, or other important areas of functioning. Chronological age is at least 5 years. The behavior is not due exclusively to the direct physiological effect of a substance or a general medical condition.	**Infancy and Early Childhood** Not relevant at this age. **Middle Childhood** The child will frequently have significant social problems and family distress related to wetting. **Adolescence** The adolescent has significant social problems, emotional difficulty, and family stress related to wetting.

SPECIAL INFORMATION
Subtypes: Nocturnal only, passage of urine only during nighttime sleep. Diurnal only, involuntary/intentional passage of urine during waking hours. Nocturnal only enuresis is the most common subtype and occurs only during nighttime sleep, typically during the first one third of the night. Nocturnal and diurnal enuresis is a combination of the two subtypes. Evaluation should determine if the wetting is primary (never had 6-month period of dryness) or secondary (wetting after at least 6 months of dryness). Approximately 75% of all children with enuresis have a first-degree biological relative who has had the disorder.

DIFFERENTIAL DIAGNOSIS	SPECIAL INFORMATION
General Medical Conditions — **Examples include:** Neurogenic bladder Urinary tract infection Spina bifida Diastematomyelia Seizure disorder Diabetes mellitus Diabetes insipidus Constipation Sleep apnea Hyperthyroidism Anatomic urologic abnormality	Urinary tract infection may be subclinical, partially treated. Constipation may be unrecognized by the family. Onset of secondary enuresis may be a first symptom of hyperthyroidism.
Substances Lithium Caffeine Theophylline Diuretics	Families may not be aware that certain foods and drinks are sources of large amounts of caffeine (e.g., in soda pop, chocolate, or iced tea).

COMMONLY COMORBID CONDITIONS	SPECIAL INFORMATION
Other Comorbid Mental Health **Conditions — Examples include:** 307.7, 787.6 Encopresis 307.46 Sleepwalking disorder 307.46 Sleep terror disorder 317, 318.x, 319 Mental retardation 315.00 Reading disorder 315.1 Mathematics disorder 315.2 Disorder of written expression	These are more likely to be associated with daytime wetting. Enuresis is rarely the only symptom of these disorders of all types that are associated with enuresis.
Other General Medical Conditions Neurologic disorders Urologic disorders Constipation Low bladder volume Inability to concentrate urine	Enuresis is rarely the only symptom of these disorders. Developmental delays of all types are associated with enuresis.

Purging/Binge Eating

Presenting Complaints

fasting

binge eating

uncontrolled eating

voluntary vomiting

laxative use

diuretic use

compulsive exercising

Definitions and Symptoms

Many preadolescents and adolescents who are concerned about their body shape and appearance use a variety of compensatory methods to prevent weight gain and eliminate unwanted calories. These methods of purging may include self-induced vomiting, ingestion of laxatives, diuretics or diet pills, compulsive exercising, and fasting. These adolescents typically purge after a binge or eating too much in a short period of time. A binge is defined as eating in a discrete period of time an amount of food that is definitely larger than most individuals would eat under similar circumstances. The individual eats with a sense of loss of control or an inability to stop eating during the binge (this is regarded as an "objective binge"). Many adolescents consider even a small amount of food, particularly foods with sugar and fat in them, to be a binge, and thus have a need to purge. It is the sense of loss of control, rather than the actual amount of food eaten, that is crucial in such cases.

Individuals who engage in binge eating and/or purging may or may not be of a normal weight. (If the individual is underweight, also consider dieting.) Whatever their actual weight, they often consider themselves too fat or perceive certain parts of their bodies (e.g., stomach, hips, or buttock) as being too big. Such body image distortions and fear of weight gain are often unrealistic compared to common growth charts or observer judgment. In some cases, parental emphasis on thinness, peer pressure, peer modeling, and/or exposure to popular media-based conceptions of a thin-normal ideal body shape may spur the development of body image distortions and the onset of dieting behavior. For preadolescents, concrete motives and beliefs such as thinking that they will be more popular and have more friends and fun if they are thinner may promote the development of body shape concerns. During puberty, the normal development of the breasts, hips, and thighs may be misinterpreted as becoming fat and lead to body image distortions. These perceived distortions are particularly problematic in gymnasts, dancers, and wrestlers.

Teenage girls are much more likely to engage in dieting behavior and have greater distortion of their body images than boys, which is consistent with the greater cultural emphasis on thinness as a measure of beauty or attractiveness for women. As a result of these distortions, the adolescent's self-evaluation is negatively influenced, resulting in low self-esteem.

Isolated episodes of purging and/or binge eating may represent a normal developmental variation because of the normative nature of concerns about body image and appearance. More frequent, intense, and regular episodes of binge eating and/or purging represent a problem. The development of a binge/purge cycle, in which the opportunity to purge facilitates the development of regular binge eating, is also a sign of a problem. There is also an increased sense of loss of control overeating, combined with more pervasive body image distortions and negative self-evaluation, at the problem level of purging/binge eating.

Epidemiology

In clinic and population samples, at least 90% of individuals with bulimia nervosa are female. The prevalence of bulimia nervosa among adolescent and young adult females is approximately 1% to 3%. The rate of occurrence in males is approximately one tenth of that in females.

DEVELOPMENTAL VARIATION	COMMON DEVELOPMENTAL PRESENTATIONS
V65.49 Purging/Binge-Eating Variation Occasional overeating or perception of overeating, either objective or subjective binges, occurs. Intermittent concern about body image or getting fat is present in specific situations during which too much food was eaten. Concerns are not pervasive or cross-situational and do not change eating behaviors. Normal weight gain is typically present.	**Infancy and Early Childhood** Not relevant at this age. **Middle Childhood** The child feels fat after eating too much at a holiday or special occasion meal, fasts or exercises, compares body shape to peers, skips a meal or two to restrain eating, may lose control when hungry and eat too much, and has a negative self-evaluation when teased or called "fat" by a peer. **Adolescence** The adolescent, as an isolated incident, purges in response to pressure from athletic coaches and/or ballet/gymnastic instructors to achieve a certain weight, or purges in imitation of peers.

PROBLEM	COMMON DEVELOPMENTAL PRESENTATIONS
V69.19 Purging/Binge-Eating Problem Includes experimentation with vomiting, laxatives, fasting, or exercises to prevent weight gain. Isolated episodes are far apart in time. Individual has increased episodes of uncontrolled eating. The individual's perceptions of body shape or size become more systematically distorted. Negative self-evaluation is often influenced by weight and body shape. The behaviors are not sufficiently intense to qualify for a diagnosis of bulimia nervosa or eating disorder, NOS.	**Infancy** Not relevant at this age. **Early Childhood** Usually not relevant at this age. **Middle Childhood** The child begins to have obsessive thoughts about how unwanted food is having an impact on body shape, body shape distortions begin to crystalize, and the child sometimes is unable to control urge to binge around certain foods, particularly when alone. **Adolescence** The adolescent vomits or uses laxatives occasionally, begins to have obsessive thoughts about how unwanted food is having an impact on body shape, has consistent body image distortions about hips, stomach, and thighs, experiences depression (see Sadness and Related Symptoms cluster, p 153), anxiety (see Anxious Symptoms cluster, p 145), conflict, and environmental stressors (see Environmental Situations Defined, p 31), or purges/binge eats as a way to meet other unmet needs.
	SPECIAL INFORMATION
	May be overweight when these behaviors begin.

223

DISORDER	COMMON DEVELOPMENTAL PRESENTATIONS
307.51 Bulimia Nervosa The essential features are recurrent episodes of binge eating and inappropriate compensatory behaviors to prevent weight gain. Recurrent episodes of binge eating and inappropriate compensatory behaviors occur at least twice a week for 3 months. Purging is accomplished through self-induced vomiting or the misuse of laxatives, diuretics, or enemas. The individual has a sense of lack of control during binge eating episodes. The person has distorted perceptions of body shape or size and may also use fasting or compulsive exercise to prevent weight gain. **307.50 Eating Disorder, Not Otherwise Specified** (see *DSM-IV* Criteria Appendix, p 327)	**Infancy and Early Childhood** Not relevant at this age. **Middle Childhood** The child primarily uses vomiting for purging, the binges may be more subjective than objective ones, is frequently influenced by peers, media, and parents, and may have a history of sexual/physical abuse (see p 45), severe psychosocial trauma (see Anxious Symptoms cluster, p 145), and severe family pathology (see Environmental Situations Defined, p 31). **Adolescence** The adolescent expands purging techniques to laxatives and other methods in addition to vomiting, acts highly secretive, eats a great deal to satisfy other unmet needs or emotions, has extremely distorted perceptions of body image or size, and exercises excessively in an attempt to compensate for binge eating.

SPECIAL INFORMATION
Middle to late adolescence is the most common age of onset. There are two subtypes of bulimia nervosa. The purging type involves regular self-induced vomiting and/or the misuse of laxatives, diuretics, or enemas. The nonpurging type involves other inappropriate compensatory behaviors, such as fasting or excessive exercise. Individuals whose binge eating/purging occurs only as part of anorexia nervosa episodes are diagnosed as having anorexia nervosa, binge-eating/purging type (see Dieting/Body Image Problems cluster, p 227). May also show impulsive behaviors such as shoplifting, promiscuity (see Secretive/Antisocial Behaviors cluster, p 127), or substance use in adolescence (see Substance Use/Abuse cluster, p 135). Families may be disengaged, highly conflictual, or even abusive (see Environmental Situations Defined, p 31).

DIFFERENTIAL DIAGNOSIS	SPECIAL INFORMATION
General Medical Conditions — Examples include: Kleine-Levin syndrome	
Substances — Examples include: Lithium Alcohol Stimulants Psychotropics	
Mental Disorders 300.4 Dysthymic disorder 307.1 Anorexia nervosa, binge-eating/ purging type 301.83 Borderline personality disorder 296.xx Major depressive disorder (with atypical features) 312.81 Conduct disorder childhood onset 312.82 Conduct disorder adolescent onset 313.81 Oppositional defiant disorder 300.02 Generalized anxiety disorder 300.3 Obsessive-compulsive disorder 309.81 Posttraumatic stress disorder	

COMMONLY COMORBID CONDITIONS	SPECIAL INFORMATION
Other Comorbid Mental Health Conditions —Examples include: **312.81** Conduct disorder childhood onset **312.82** Conduct disorder adolescent onset **313.81** Oppositional defiant disorder **300.02** Generalized anxiety disorder **309.81** Posttraumatic stress disorder **309.21** Separation anxiety disorder **314.xx** Attention-deficit/hyperactivity disorder **296.2x, 296.3x** Major depressive disorder **300.4** Dysthymic disorder **305** Substance abuse or dependence **301.83** Borderline personality disorder **300.3** Obsessive-compulsive disorder **296** Bipolar disorder	Individuals with bulimia nervosa typically are within the normal weight range, although some may be slightly overweight or underweight.
Other General Medical Conditions — Examples include: Dental problems Enlarged salivary glands Calluses or scars on dorsal surface of hand Cardiac and skeletal myopathies Menstrual irregularity or amenorrhea Fluid and electrolyte disturbances Esophageal tears, gastric rupture, and cardiac arrhythmias Diabetes mellitus	Patients with bulimia experience a loss of dental enamel and increased frequency of dental cavities due to recurrent vomiting. Serious cardiac and skeletal myopathies result from regular use of syrup of ipecac to induce vomiting. Rare but potentially fatal complications include esophageal tears, gastric rupture, and cardiac arrhythmias. Individuals who chronically abuse laxatives may become dependent on their use to stimulate bowel movements.

Presenting Complaints

dieting
losing weight
restricting food intake
disturbance in perception of body shape or size
afraid of getting fat

Definitions and Symptoms

Many adolescents and preadolescents diet, voluntarily restricting their food intake in order to lose weight. They often start dieting because they think they are too fat or perceive certain parts of their body (e.g., stomach, hips, or buttocks) as being too big. Such perceptions of becoming fat are often unrealistic or distorted compared to common growth charts or observer judgment.

In some cases, primarily in adolescents, peer pressure, parental emphasis on thinness, pressure from coaches to be at a certain weight or attain a certain appearance, and/or exposure to popular media-based conceptions of an ideal body shape may spur the development of body image distortions and the onset of dieting behavior. In other cases, primarily in middle childhood, restricting food intake is less often associated with body image distortions and more often associated with concrete phobias (fear of choking, food contamination, fear of growing up), specific beliefs (thinness will lead to popularity and more friends), and family conflicts over control issues. Teenage girls are much more likely to engage in dieting behavior and have body image disturbances than boys, which is consistent with the greater cultural emphasis on thinness as a measure of beauty or attractiveness for women.

Although some dieting behavior and overconcern about body shape are normative during adolescence, some teenagers engage in these behaviors to the point of endangering their physical and mental health. The normative dieting and body shape concerns of adolescence become a problem when the adolescent meets at least one of the following conditions: 1) restricts food intake to the point where body weight consistently stays below normal, 2) obsessively pursues thinness and fears fatness, 3) consistently has a distorted perception of body shape or size, and/ or 4) has irregular menstruation, with no prior menstrual abnormalities for medical reasons. Denial of dieting also commonly starts to be a problem at this stage. When body weight drops at least 15% below normal and all of the other previously mentioned conditions apply, a dieting/ body image problem becomes the syndrome of anorexia nervosa. (The term anorexia is a misnomer because loss of appetite is rare.) It is important to consider the individual's body build and weight history in determining minimally normal weight.

Epidemiology

Prevalence studies among females in late adolescence and early adulthood have found rates of 0.5% to 1.0% for presentations that meet full criteria for anorexia nervosa. Its incidence has been increasing in recent decades. The onset is often associated with a stressful life/family event or physical illness resulting in mild weight loss. Individuals who are subthreshold for the disorder (at the problem level) are more commonly encountered. More than 90% of cases occur in women. Anorexia nervosa is more common among middle and upper socioeconomic status and in industrialized countries. The most common age of onset is 14 to 15 years, in early adolescence.

Of individuals admitted to university hospitals, the death rate from anorexia nervosa is approximately 10%, usually due to electrolyte imbalance, starvation, suicide, cardiac arrhythmia, or congestive heart failure.

Anorexia nervosa may be the restricting type, in which binge eating or purging is not present during the current episode, or the binge-eating/purging type, in which binge eating or purging occurs during the current episode.

DEVELOPMENTAL VARIATION	COMMON DEVELOPMENTAL PRESENTATIONS
V65.49 Dieting/Body Image Variation Dieting may occur if the child is overweight but it should be a realistic program. The child does not completely eliminate any food group, but generally decreases intake of food, especially of sweets and fats or is on an appropriate diet. The child favors a thin appearance but has a realistic image. The individual can stop dieting voluntarily.	**Infancy** Not relevant at this age. **Early Childhood** In early childhood, children usually do not restrict food for dieting purposes, but they may develop a fear of specific foods or food aversions. **Middle Childhood** The child may have short attempts at dieting with minimal or appropriate weight loss, skips deserts and snacks, occasionally throws out lunch in school, experiences peer pressure and modeling as major factors, and tries to diet after being teased about being fat by a peer. **Adolescence** The adolescent does not eat red meat, sweets, and fats, or skips meals. The adolescent is highly responsive to peer or media pressure, diets to look good to attract a sexual partner, systematically uses exercise to lose weight.
	SPECIAL INFORMATION
	Adolescence is the common age of onset of serious dieting. Constipation can cause a decrease in appetite at all ages.

PROBLEM	COMMON DEVELOPMENTAL PRESENTATIONS
V69.1 Dieting/Body Image Problem Dieting and voluntary food restrictions are more restrictive and result in weight loss or failure to gain weight as expected during growth but these behaviors are not sufficiently intense to qualify for the diagnosis of anorexia nervosa or eating disorder, NOS. The individual begins to become obsessed with the pursuit of thinness and develops systematic fears of gaining weight. The individual also begins to develop a consistent disturbance in body perception and starts to deny that weight loss or dieting is a problem.	**Infancy and Early Childhood** Not relevant at this age. **Middle Childhood** The child may occasionally diet inappropriately, fails to grow as expected (more common than actual weight loss), or often develops this problem under pressure from coaches in competitive athletics, skating, dancing, or other hobbies in which thinness is important. **Adolescence** The adolescent starts skipping meals for a brief period of time, fasts, eliminates entire food groups (e.g., fats or sweets), may become overly focused on food, cooking, and shopping but refuses to eat, has a change in eating habits — takes small bites, dawdles at meals, has ritualistic beliefs about food (e.g., one cookie leads to weight gain), gets full fast as stomach shrinks from weight loss, may interpret fullness as fatness, sees specific body parts (abdomen, hips, and thighs) as too large, views menstrual irregularity as positive (i.e., wants to be like a little girl), and begins to deny that weight beliefs and eating are problems. Adolescents engaging in this behavior are often involved in highly competitive sports or artistic endeavors (e.g., ballet, skating, or gymnastics).

SPECIAL INFORMATION
Families may be overly involved, overprotective, high achieving, perfectionistic, overly compliant, and high approval-seeking (see Environmental Situations Defined, p 31). Parents often show difficulty with adolescent individualization. Adolescents often have extreme self-discipline in many areas of their lives.

DISORDER	COMMON DEVELOPMENTAL PRESENTATIONS
307.1 Anorexia Nervosa Refusal to maintain body weight at or above minimally normal weight for age and height. Weight loss leads to body weight being maintained at less than 85% of that expected. Body mass index (weight in kilograms divided by [height in meters]²) is 17.5 kg/m² for older adolescents. Use body mass index tables for middle childhood and early adolescence. Failure to gain weight during growth results in body weight being maintained at less than 85% of that expected. The individual intensely fears gaining weight or becoming fat, experiences a disturbance in the way in which one's body shape or size is experienced, and denies the seriousness of weight loss or a low body weight. In postmenarcheal girls, amenorrhea (i.e., the absence of at least three consecutive menstrual cycles). There are a number of different methods that may be used to evaluate whether the individual's weight is below the minimally normal level. Always consider the individual's body build and weight history.	**Infancy and Early Childhood** Usually not relevant. **Middle Childhood** The child diets, fails to gain weight as expected (more common than weight loss), has concrete fears more common than fear of gaining weight, often does not verbalize fears or distortions in perception of body shape/size; clinicians often discover these phenomena when the children are asked to eat more and gain weight. The child may begin to exercise excessively. **Adolescence** The adolescent may chronically diet, has loss of menses, has distorted body image, fears gaining weight or becoming fat even though underweight, compulsively exercises, is moody and irritable, withdraws from peers and parents, is often overly compliant in all areas but eating, expresses extreme denial of the problem, and is preoccupied with thoughts of food. The adolescent exercises to control or lose weight.

	SPECIAL INFORMATION
307.5 Eating Disorder, Not Otherwise Specified (see *DSM-IV* Criteria Appendix, p 327)	Consider the individual's body build and weight history in determining minimally normal weight. Anorexia nervosa is more common among those of middle and upper socioeconomic status and in industrialized nations. Of individuals admitted to university hospitals, the death rate in anorexia nervosa is approximately 10%, usually due to electrolyte imbalance, starvation, suicide, cardiac arrhythmia, or congestive heart failure. Anorexia nervosa may be the restricting type, in which binge eating or purging does not occur during the current episode, or the binge-eating/purging type, in which binge eating or purging occurs during the current episode. The onset is often associated with a stressful life/family event (see Environmental Situations Defined, p 31) or physical illness resulting in mild weight loss. Severe anorexia nervosa, with onset before puberty, may permanently alter full development of secondary sexual characteristics and sometimes is associated with persistent amenorrhea, even after recovery of a normal body weight.

DIFFERENTIAL DIAGNOSIS	SPECIAL INFORMATION
General Medical Conditions — **Examples include:** Chronic illness Gastrointestinal disease Brain tumors Occult malignancies Acquired immunodeficiency syndrome Tuberculosis Superior mesenteric artery syndrome Addison's disease Diabetes mellitus or insipidus Hypothyroidism/hyperthyroidism	Patients with Addison's disease have an increased heart rate; patients with anorexia nervosa have a decreased heart rate. Distortion of body image will not likely be present.
Substances — Examples include: Cocaine Amphetamines Methylphenidate	Weight loss may occur but there will not be the presence of a distorted body image.
Mental Disorders **300.4** Dysthymia **296.2x,** Major depressive disorder **296.3x** **295.xx** Schizophrenia **300.23** Social phobia **300.3** Obsessive-compulsive disorder **300.7** Body dysmorphic disorder **307.51** Bulimia nervosa **300.82** Somatization **296.xx** Bipolar disorder **309.81** Posttraumatic stress disorder **300.xx** Anxiety disorders	

COMMONLY COMORBID CONDITIONS	SPECIAL INFORMATION
Other Comorbid Mental Health Conditions — Examples include: **296.2x,** Major depressive disorder **296.3x** **300.3** Obsessive-compulsive disorder **300.xx** Anxiety disorder	Distinguish between depressed affect secondary to starvation and major depressive disorder (see Sadness and Related Symptoms cluster, p 153). When individuals with anorexia nervosa exhibit obsessions and compulsions that are not related to food, body shape, or weight, an additional diagnosis of obsessive-compulsive disorder may be warranted (see Ritualistic, Obsessive, Compulsive Symptoms cluster, p 161).
Other General Medical Conditions Scars and calluses on the dorsum of the hand Hypertrophy of the salivary glands Hypercarotenemia Peripheral edema Bradycardia, cardiac arrhythmias Lanugo Amenorrhea Constipation Cold intolerance Lethargy Excess energy Emaciation Hypotension Hypothermia Dryness of skin Hypothermic/pituitary dysfunction Liver function abnormalities Leukopenia Thrombocytopenia Electrolyte imbalance	Semistarvation of anorexia nervosa, and the purging behaviors sometimes associated with it, can result in the development of normochromic normocytic anemia, impaired renal function, cardio-vascular problems, dental problems, and osteoporosis.

Presenting Complaints

poor appetite

failure to thrive

finicky eating

poor weight gain

excessive appetite

excessive weight gain

excess nutritional intake

obesity

Definitions and Symptoms

The eating disorders cluster is characterized by disturbances in eating behaviors, several of which can be clinically severe. Although the Eating Disorders section in *DSM-IV* is focused on severe disturbances of eating behavior, the primary care physician is much more frequently concerned with the range of normal eating behaviors in infants, children, and adolescents. Parents are frequently concerned that their children are eating inadequately, eating improperly, or are not gaining enough weight. Surprisingly, issues concerning excessive weight gain are less frequently brought to the physician's attention. Although parents may not be concerned about their children being overweight, the problem of being overweight frequently becomes important for children in middle childhood or adolescence. However, longitudinal studies relating childhood obesity to adult mortality are rare.

The diagnosis of feeding disorder of infancy or early childhood is of particular concern to pediatric clinicians treating those in infancy and early childhood. The diagnosis, used to describe infants and young children whose weight is consistently below the 5th percentile curve or who show accelerated decrease in growth velocity in the absence of constitutional delay, has been traditionally divided into organic and nonorganic forms. The inclusion of an interactional or mixed category encompassing both types is necessary in a large percentage of cases.

Etiology

In reviewing eating and nutritional concerns, it is critical to consider whether or not a lack of resources, knowledge, or parental understanding may be playing a role in an individual patient's clinical situation.

Epidemiology

Of all pediatric hospital admissions, 1% to 5% are for failure to gain adequate weight, and up to half of these may reflect feeding disturbances without any apparent predisposing general medical condition.

DEVELOPMENTAL VARIATION	COMMON DEVELOPMENTAL PRESENTATIONS
V65.49 Inadequate Nutrition Variation The individual has less than average nutritional intake for age, but is within 3% of normal growth for height and weight. The individual has growth weight and height <30th percentile — without constitutional cause.	**Infancy** The child is a finicky eater and spits. Vomiting may be due to overfeeding. **Early and Middle Childhood** The child has a poor appetite and is a finicky eater. Children who grow rapidly and attain early increased stature frequently do so on a constitutional or genetic basis. **Adolescence** The adolescent is a finicky eater, concerned about weight and body image, and has food fads/food preferences, or is swayed by foods eaten by peers.
	SPECIAL INFORMATION
	Genetic factors have a significant role in the ultimate growth pattern of a child. Intercurrent family, social, financial, medical, or psychological issues may interfere with a mother's ability to nourish her child. Determination of the caregiver's child rearing beliefs is critical. Children with irregular temperament may at times refuse meals.

DEVELOPMENTAL VARIATION	COMMON DEVELOPMENTAL PRESENTATIONS
V65.4 Excessive Nutrition Intake Variation The individual appears to eat a great deal but has a normal growth rate.	**Infancy** The child eats eagerly and frequently seems hungry. **Early Childhood** The child overeats certain foods and clearly has food preferences. Appetite frequently decreases dramatically between ages 1 and 2. **Middle Childhood and Adolescence** The child or adolescent overeats certain foods and has strong food preferences. Eating during periods of growth spurts may appear excessive.
	SPECIAL INFORMATION
	See a growth chart for median growth information.

PROBLEM	COMMON DEVELOPMENTAL PRESENTATIONS
V40.3 Inadequate Nutrition Intake Problem Individual fails to grow in a normal fashion and fails to maintain growth velocity. Growth is at or below 3% for height and weight for more than 6 months. Protein-calorie malnutrition reflects inadequate intake, excessive losses, or excessive calorie utilization.	**Infancy** The infant may have food refusals. Associated with this, the infant may have low oral-motor tone, oversensitivity to certain textures, or a reduced ability to taste. **Early Childhood** The child's negative behaviors involving increasing independence may result in refusal to eat. Classically this is known as a problem of individuation or an oppositional feeding problem. Children with oppositional feeding problem are at risk for inadequate growth due to rejection of oral intake. Children with sensory integration problems have associated tactile defensiveness that can also lead to inadequate nutrition. Parents may be uncomfortable with their children feeding themselves. **Middle Childhood and Adolescence** Since older children are more independent in their ability to obtain and eat food, inadequate eating is most likely associated with perceived need to diet (see Diet/Body Image cluster, p 227).

SPECIAL INFORMATION
Consider inadequate resources, incorrect nutritional information, poor feeding technique, or stressful or conflicted feedings. After the infant's first year of life, breast milk should not be viewed as the major nutritional source. Breastfeeding failure rates are higher in mother-child pairs living in isolation with a low income or educational level and who participate in government poverty programs. Some infants have difficulties with homeostasis — they are unable to sense their own hunger, never become satisfied, and experience disruption of the normal hunger-satisfy cycle. Families concerned about arteriosclerotic heart disease may inappropriately provide an infant with skim milk. Confusion may exist concerning the use of soy formula (nutritionally complete formula) versus soy milk. Parents who are vegetarians may feed an infant a diet that is inadequate in protein.

PROBLEM	COMMON DEVELOPMENTAL PRESENTATIONS
V40.3 Excessive Nutrition Intake Problem The individual has a caloric intake greater than the number of calories necessary to allow for normal growth. (When tricep skinfold thickness is in excess of 85% it constitutes obesity.)	**Infancy** The child is overfed by parents and misunderstands cues. Associated with this, the infant may have low oral-motor tone, oversensitivity to certain textures, or a reduced ability to taste. **Early Childhood** The child overeats preferred food and continually asks for more. **Middle Childhood** The child overeats, steals or sneaks food, and has decreased physical activity. **Adolescence** The adolescent who overeats may be resistant to eating low-calorie foods, snacks frequently, and usually has decreased physical activity.

	SPECIAL INFORMATION
	Consider lifestyle issues (overscheduling, overeating of fast food). Consider the use of food as a bribe or reward. Increased food intake is associated with watching television. Watching television for more than 3 to 4 hours a day is associated with an increase in childhood obesity probably secondary to decreased activity combined with excessive intake. Obese children are taller and tend to have advanced bone ages when compared to nonobese peers. It is important to distinguish children who are overweight from those who are overfat. Children whose weight exceeds 120% of their expected weight should be defined as overfat. Parental focus on a child who is overweight but not overfat contributes to an inappropriate body image focus. Both hereditary and environmental issues can have a significant association with obesity. Parental obesity, high socioeconomic class, smaller family size, and parental education beyond high school are positively associated with childhood obesity. Consider peer pressure, low self-esteem, and death of a family member as part of the diagnosis. Onset of obesity during adolescence has a higher potential for body image issues. Dissatisfaction with body shape or size is more common in females than in males and in whites than in African-Americans. Both obese and nonobese adolescents underreport their dietary intake. Increased fat intake is strongly related to obesity and reduction in fat intake is associated with obesity prevention. The two most common measures of adiposity are the body mass index and triceps skinfold measurement. Body mass index is weight measured in kilograms divided by height in square meters. Triceps skinfold thickness is the width of the subcutaneous fat over the triceps muscle measured midway between the olecranon process and the acromioclavicular joint.

DISORDER	COMMON DEVELOPMENTAL PRESENTATIONS
307.59 Feeding Disorder of Infancy or Early Childhood This disorder involves a feeding disturbance between parent and child as manifested by a persistent failure to eat adequately with a significant failure to gain weight or loss of a significant amount of weight over at least 1 month. The disturbance is not due to an associated gastrointestinal or other general medical condition. The disturbance is not better accounted for by another mental disorder or by lack of available food. The onset is before age 6 years.	**Infancy** The infant fails to gain weight adequately. The infant loses weight over a period of at least 1 month. Associated findings include deficient sleep and bowel disorders. Associated with this, the infant may have low oral-motor tone, oversensitivity to certain textures, or a reduced ability to taste. **Early Childhood** The child refuses/fails to eat adequately and fails to gain weight or loses weight over a period of at least 1 month.
	SPECIAL INFORMATION
	Nonorganic risk factors for feeding disorder of infancy and childhood include difficult temperament, disturbed interactions with caregiver (see p 45), aversive feeding behavior in the child, and familial psychosocial stressors (see p 45). Infants who are developmentally and physically immature, withdrawn, or lethargic are at increased risk for feeding problems. Additional risk factors include problems of attachment, autonomy, self-regulation, and separation.

DIFFERENTIAL DIAGNOSIS	SPECIAL INFORMATION
General Medical Conditions — Examples include:	Consider inflammatory bowel disease when decreased weight and appetite are abrupt.
Inadequate intake	Increased calorie utilization occurs from increased motor activity, intercurrent acute illness, or recurrent febrile illnesses.
Urinary tract infections	An increased amount of breathing and sucking in chronic cardiac respiratory illness tends to account for decreased growth.
Renal tubular acidosis	
Chronic renal failure	Primary obesity is associated with increased height, bone age, and early menses. Most genetic syndromes associated with obesity have short stature, delayed bone age, and delayed secondary sexual characteristics.
Thyroid pituitary disease	
Congenital heart disease	
Sugar intolerance	
Gastroesophageal reflux	
Chromosomal abnormality	
Lead toxicity	
Pregnancy	
Milk/soy allergy	
Tuberculosis	
Constipation	
Cystic fibrosis	
Inflammatory bowel disease	
Chronic liver disease	
Neurological condition	
Diabetes mellitus	
Malnutrition	
Human immunodeficiency virus infection	
Congenital intrauterine growth retardation	
Acute neonatal hyperthyroidism	
Celiac disease	
Iron, zinc deficiency	
Excessive intake	
Laurence-Moon-Biedl syndrome	
Turner syndrome	
Mucopolysaccharidosis	
Endocrinology condition	
Cushing syndrome	
Hypothalamic lesions	
Glycogen storage disease	
Hypothyroidism	
Beckwith syndrome	
Prader-Willi syndrome	

DIFFERENTIAL DIAGNOSIS, CONTINUED	SPECIAL INFORMATION, CONTINUED
Substances — Examples include: *Inadequate intake* Antibiotics Diphenylhydantoin Methylphenidate Amphetamines Digitalis Pemoline Antimetabolites Ephedrine Cocaine Cancer chemotherapeutic agents Cigarette smoking *Excessive intake* Phenothiazines Corticosteroids Marijuana Lithium Clonidine Tricyclics	Therapies for a chronic medical condition can decrease food intake.
Mental Disorders **307.52** Pica **307.53** Rumination disorder **317,** Mental retardation **318.x,** **319** **309.21** Separation anxiety disorder	

COMMONLY COMORBID CONDITIONS	SPECIAL INFORMATION
Other Comorbid Mental Health Conditions — Examples include: *Inadequate intake* **300.02** Generalized anxiety disorder **309.81** Posttraumatic stress disorder **309.21** Separation anxiety disorder **295.xx** Schizophrenia **300.3** Obsessive-compulsive disorder **299.00** Autistic disorder **296.2x,** Major depressive disorder **298.3x** **313.89** Reactive attachment disorder **300.4** Dysthymic disorder Heightened family tension around mealtime (stressor) *Excessive intake - stressors*	Infants with feeding disorders are often especially irritable and difficult to console during feeding. Inadequate caloric intake may exacerbate the associated features (irritability, developmental lags) and further contribute to feeding difficulties. Other associated conditions include neuroregulatory difficulties and preexisting developmental impairments. Other factors that may be associated with the condition include parental psychopathology and child abuse or neglect (see p 45). Children associate obesity with a variety of negative stereotypes. Obesity has been associated with decreased acceptance rates into college, lower social class, and decreased employability. Obese children are frequently ridiculed, and they often seek younger children as friends. Obesity may lead to overestimates of age and inappropriate behavioral expectations. Family members can be particularly resistant to having children deal with the issue of being overweight (the "food is love" phenomenon). An associated feature may include heightened family tension around mealtime. In the pervasive developmental disorders (see Social Interaction Behaviors cluster, p 277), there may be associated eating abnormalities such as the child's diet is limited to a very few foods, excessive fluid intake, and exaggerated reactions to food odors.
Other General Medical Conditions *Inadequate intake* Fragile X syndrome Tactile defensiveness Oral-motor dysfunction Cleft lip/palate Pregnancy *Excessive intake* Early menarche Precocious puberty Cardiovascular or pulmonary complications leading to increased mortality as adults	Early menarche in an obese female may be confused with premature puberty.

ILLNESS-RELATED BEHAVIORS

PSYCHOLOGICAL FACTORS AFFECTING MEDICAL CONDITION

PSYCHOLOGICAL FACTORS AFFECTING MEDICAL CONDITION

Presenting Complaints

inappropriate behaviors related to health care experiences

problems with use of services or adherence to medical
    regimen

precociously mature attitudes and/or behaviors toward
    illness

denial of importance or severity of illness

Definitions and Symptoms

The essential feature of psychological factors affecting medical condition is the presence of one or more specific psychological or behavioral factors that adversely affect a general medical condition. These factors include mental disorders, psychological symptoms, personality traits or coping style, maladaptive health behaviors, stress-related physiological responses, and/or other or unspecified factors.

Health-related behaviors refer to behaviors associated with a medical condition and/or its treatment that have their origin in the illness or disability experience. Some health-related behaviors may be adaptive and can be anticipated in almost any childhood illness experience. Psychological factors such as coping style may also affect health-related behaviors. Family factors are often extremely important and may interrelate with health-related behaviors. *Developmental variations* consist of occasional inappropriate behaviors designed to influence events, especially treatment. In the adolescent, these variations may manifest themselves in use of services or treatment adherence. Normal developmental variations have a minimal effect on the child's health or well-being. *Behaviors at the problem level* are characterized by frequent inappropriate health-related behaviors, manipulation of the health care system, frequent underadherence or overadherence to treatment, or ignoring risk factors known to cause or exacerbate the medical condition but behaviors are not sufficiently intense to qualify for the diagnosis of *psychological factors affecting medical condition. A disorder* consists of behaviors so persistent and inappropriate that they can pose a severe risk to the child's health or well-being, especially in the adolescent, who is capable of largely autonomous activity. In the primary care setting, this child may be identified by his or her bargaining or negotiation, or preference for certain events around treatments that range from expected adaptation to behaviors sufficiently persistent and problematic to pose severe risk or actual injury. The provider's concern regarding maladaptive health-related behaviors should be related to their persistence and the level of risk they present to the child's health and well-being. The diagnostic category at the disorder level for this cluster is not a true disorder in the *DSM-IV* classification system, but *psychological factors affecting medical condition* best represents the category for this cluster.

Primary Care Presentation

Pseudomaturity refers to a child's use of coping strategies that are excessively mature for the child's expected developmental stage. Some pseudomaturity may be normal and adaptive in acute or chronic illness. Occasional displays of inappropriately mature behavior that do not interfere with function and/or relationships may be a developmental variation. Moderately frequent behavior associated with precocious responsibility and some interference with functioning can be categorized as a problem. The child's behavior may be too cautious, hyper-responsible, and intellectualized. The child may display limited or no emotions, but consistently demonstrates precocious self-management in areas related to the illness and other aspects of life.

Denial, in this context, is the inability or refusal to accept or acknowledge the reality or significance of medical conditions or symptoms in a manner that compromises adaptation or puts health status at risk. Denial arises from the need to reduce overwhelming anxiety by ignoring or avoiding the recognition of reality that is too emotionally painful or distressing. At times denial may have adaptive qualities by allowing a person to avoid preoccupation with illness by not focusing on it for extended periods. Serious mental disorders can be distinguished because they predate the health condition and/or affect many areas of the child's functioning and have symptoms characteristic of the disorder.

DEVELOPMENTAL VARIATION	COMMON DEVELOPMENTAL PRESENTATIONS
V65.49 Health-Related Behaviors Variation Occasional health-related behaviors occur that pose little or no risk to the child's health or well-being. The child may display occasional or limited pseudomaturity that causes little or no interference with age-appropriate functioning and relationships. Denial may take the form of a simple refusal to admit to or acknowledge physical symptoms or a loss of function. The child may become distant or detached during attempts to discuss or treat the condition. Among adolescents, denial may take an intellectualized form in which efforts are made to disprove or explain away the symptoms in an unrealistic manner.	**Infancy** The infant sometimes does not find physical examinations pleasant and may cry. **Early Childhood** The child bargains or negotiates for certain treatments (e.g., oral treatments as opposed to injections) and uses simple denial ("I'm not sick"). **Middle Childhood** The child bargains or negotiates preferences for certain events around treatment, wants to be in charge of medication, occasionally uses sophisticated medical terms, and uses simple denial, or may use magical thinking ("I'll get better"). **Adolescence** The adolescent varies patterns of use of health care services or degree of adherence to regimen, and uses simple to more complex denial when facts cannot be fully comprehended ("I can prove I'm not sick"). The adolescent may not take medications on time.
	SPECIAL INFORMATION
	Some health-related behaviors may be normal and adaptive in acute or chronic illnesses. Some denial is consistent with adaptation, when it prevents individuals from becoming preoccupied with the illness by "not thinking about it."

PROBLEM	COMMON DEVELOPMENTAL PRESENTATIONS
V15.81 Health-Related Behaviors Problem Frequent health-related behaviors occur that begin to pose a risk to the child's health or well-being. The child or caregiver may neglect prescribed treatment or make inappropriate substitutions in care plans. Such behaviors reflect a lack of awareness of the validity of the treatment plan or refusal to believe the diagnosis or prognosis. With *pseudomaturity*, the child may display mature behaviors that begin to interfere with functioning or relationships. These behaviors are not sufficiently intense to qualify for the diagnosis of psychological factors affecting medical conditions.	**Infancy** The infant cries and is noncompliant when examined but can be consoled and the examination can be completed. **Early Childhood** The child frequently engages in problematic bargaining or negotiating and clearly prefers certain events around treatment. The child often appears too serious/not playful, and often uses simple nonadaptive refusal ("I don't need it; I don't want it"). **Middle Childhood** The child frequently takes too much responsibility for aspects of care and demonstrates pseudomature behavior that makes it difficult to play with peers. The child has difficulty playing with peers of his or her own age, often engages in problematic bargaining or negotiation, and prefers one treatment over others. The child uses simple nonadaptive refusal ("I don't need it; I don't want it"). **Adolescence** The adolescent uses health care services inappropriately, does not adhere to a treatment regimen, interacts mainly with adults, engages in few age-appropriate activities/relationships, fails to comply and appear for appointments, and uses simple nonadaptive refusal to the extent that it begins to have a significant impact on the effectiveness of treatment.
	SPECIAL INFORMATION
	Frequent inappropriate, health-seeking behavior is seen, with manipulation of the health care system or frequent underadherence or overadherence to the treatment regimen. Denial may lead individuals or families to not comply with or refuse treatment. Cultural beliefs may lead to culturally based refusal of treatment that reflects special interpretations of the illness and treatment. It is important to consider health-related situations.

DISORDER	COMMON DEVELOPMENTAL PRESENTATIONS
316 Psychological Factors Affecting Medical Condition Psychological factors that affect the general medical condition by: influencing the course of their general medical condition, interfering with the treatment of the medical condition, causing an additional health risk for the individual, or stress responses precipitating or exacerbating symptoms of the medical condition.	**Infancy** The infant becomes agitated and cries when in a medical setting. It becomes extremely difficult to obtain an adequate examination. **Early Childhood** The child engages in markedly inappropriate problematic bargaining or negotiation for certain treatments, consistently appears too serious/not playful, and refuses to accept parental guidance. **Middle Childhood** The child shows a marked preference for certain treatments, tries to control care to the extent that medical safety is compromised, has a consistently serious demeanor and language, refuses to participate in age-appropriate activities, and insists that others do things his or her way. **Adolescence** The adolescent does not adhere to treatment program, uses health care services inappropriately, assumes all decision making about illness management, makes errors in judgment that may result in severe health consequences, takes excessive risks, and denies the significance of illness.
	SPECIAL INFORMATION
	Persistent or prolonged inappropriate health-seeking behavior is seen with manipulation of the health care system or a persistent pattern of underadherence or overadherence to the treatment regimen. It is important to consider health-related situations.

DIFFERENTIAL DIAGNOSIS	SPECIAL INFORMATION
General Medical Conditions — **Examples include:** Focal neurologic lesions (frontal, tempo- ral, midline) Seizure epiphenomena (behavior changes related to seizure activity) Tourette's disorder Degenerative neurologic conditions (leukodystrophy) Degenerative metabolic disease	Any medical condition that results in impairment of judgment, memory, orientation, cognition, or misinterpretation of social situations may appear to be a health-related behavior problem.
Substances — Examples include: Alcohol Illegal/street drugs Prescribed medications (steroids, seda- tives, anticonvulsants, antihistamines)	Substance abuse (see Substance Use/Abuse cluster, p 135) could negatively affect the use of health care services, manipulation of the health care system, and degree of adherence to a treatment regimen. Alterations in consciousness may lead to denial.
Mental Disorders **294.xx** Dementia	Most mental disorders with the exception of those that significantly impair cognition (e.g., mental retardation and autism) can cause compliance problems with treatment. If a disorder is present, code the disorder. These conditions are likely to be manifestations of or reactions to the child's experience of illness and/or treatment. Pseudomaturity associated with environment factors may include parental unavailability, parental immaturity, parent/child role reversal (see other relationship problems, p 45), severity of illness, behaviors endorsed by caregivers, or assumption or assignment of blame. Cultural factors may affect a nonpsychiatric medical condition.

COMMONLY COMORBID CONDITIONS	SPECIAL INFORMATION
Other Comorbid Mental Health Conditions Not relevant.	
Other General Medical Conditions Not relevant.	

SEXUAL BEHAVIORS

GENDER IDENTITY ISSUES

SEXUAL DEVELOPMENT BEHAVIORS

Presenting Complaints

wishing to be the other gender

insisting that one is the other gender

persistent cross-dressing

persistent stereotypical cross-gender preferences

discomfort with one's sexual anatomy

Definitions and Symptoms

Gender identity refers to one's knowledge that one belongs to the category of male or female and to one's sense of self as male or female. Sexual identity refers to one's identification with sexual attraction to the same or other sex. This section primarily addresses gender identity problems, not sexual identity issues. Problems in gender identity development are characterized by a persistent pattern of extensive stereotypical cross-gender behavior. Boys may manifest a preference for dressing in girls' or women's clothes, playing stereotypical girls' games, playing house, drawing pictures of beautiful girls and princesses, and watching television/videos of their favorite female characters. Stereotypical female-type dolls, such as Barbie, are often their favorite toys and girls are their preferred playmates. These boys role-play female figures when playing house and avoid rough-and-tumble play and competitive sports. They have little interest in cars and trucks or other nonaggressive but stereotypical boys' toys. The boys may insist on sitting to urinate. Girls with gender identity disorder display intense negative reactions to wearing feminine attire. They prefer boys' clothes and short hair. Their fantasy heroes are most often powerful male figures. These girls show little interest in dolls and feminine dress-up or role-play activity. Cross-dressing, cross-gender role play, and cross-gender toy play often occur together with the stated desire to become a member of the other sex. Some youngsters with this problem also express dislike about their sexual anatomy. The display of periodic or transient cross-gender behaviors, however, is not uncommon, particularly during toddlerhood and early childhood. Thus, isolated or infrequent displays of cross-gender behavior are usually not of clinical concern.

Children with gender identity problems often have other difficulties in their psychosocial development. In boys, emotional problems, such as separation anxiety (see Anxious Symptoms cluster, p 145), depression (see Sadness and Related Symptoms cluster, p 153), and social withdrawal are common. These problems are related to several factors, including family difficulties and marital conflict (see p 44), parental stress, parental mental disorders (see p 46), and social ostracism. Similar problems have been noted for girls with gender identity conflict, although the greater societal acceptance of cross-gender behavior in girls sometimes results in a tendency to overlook the internal conflict girls may experience.

Because gender identity formation typically consolidates between the second and fourth years of life, the presence of extensive cross-gender behavior during this developmental period should be carefully evaluated. During childhood, the most important sequelae of gender identity conflict include poor self-esteem and alienation from the peer group. If gender identity conflict during childhood persists, the risk increases that during adolescence some of these youngsters will seek out hormonal and physical sex-modifying procedures, commonly called sex-reassignment surgery. Adult homosexuality is very rarely associated with any gender identity disorder although adults who identify themselves as homosexuals often have had some gender atypical interests (e.g., toys, activities) in their childhood histories.

Epidemiology

The prevalence of gender identity problems in children is unknown, but the general consensus is that they are relatively uncommon. A key diagnostic issue is the frequency, intensity, and duration of a variety of cross-gender behaviors. Parents often seek professional advice after their child has been manifesting such behaviors for several months or longer.

DEVELOPMENTAL VARIATION	COMMON DEVELOPMENTAL PRESENTATIONS
V65.49 Cross-Gender Behavior Variation On average, boys and girls display gender-typical preferences and behaviors. Isolated or transient cross-gender behaviors are not uncommon, particularly during toddlerhood and early childhood. Thus, isolated or transient stereotypical cross-gender behavior is usually not of clinical concern.	**Infancy** Not relevant at this age. **Early Childhood** In early childhood, the child may occasionally cross-dress, engage in cross-gender role play, toy play, and peer play. **Middle Childhood** The child may occasionally cross-dress, engage in cross-gender role play, toy play, and peer play. **Adolescence** The adolescent may occasionally cross-dress as a form of play and may have some atypical cross-gender interests.

SPECIAL INFORMATION
During early childhood, cross-gender behavior may occur briefly following a stressful life event (see p 31). For example, after the birth of a sister, a little boy might express the wish to be a girl, but this dissipates rapidly with parental support. Young children, even after they begin to understand the anatomical distinctions between the sexes, may on occasion express the desire to have attributes of the other sex (e.g., in girls, a penis; in boys, the desire to give birth to a baby). This only has significance in terms of gender identity conflict if it is occurring in the context of pervasive and persistent stereotypical cross-gender interests that is accompanied by a dislike of or discomfort with being their own sex.

PROBLEM	COMMON DEVELOPMENTAL PRESENTATIONS
V40.3 Cross-Gender Behavior Problem Usually boys and girls display gender-typical preferences and behaviors. At the problem level, the display of periodic cross-gender behaviors is more persistent and the child is notably different from same-sex peers but the behaviors are not sufficiently intense to qualify for childhood on adolescent gender identity disorders.	**Infancy** Boys repeatedly show a strong interest in their mother's clothing (e.g., walking in high heels) beginning at around 18 to 24 months of age. **Early Childhood** The child occasionally cross-dresses, engages in cross-gender role play, toy play, and peer play that persists over a period of 6 months, periodically states that he or she would like to become a member of the opposite sex, does not show an interest in sex-typical behaviors, including playing with same-sex peers, emulation of same-sex fantasy models, and same-sex toy and activity interests or the desire to have anatomic appendages of the opposite sex. **Middle Childhood** The child occasionally cross-dresses, engages in stereotypical cross-gender role play, toy play, and peer play that persists over a period of 6 months, periodically states that he or she would like to become a member of the other sex, does not show an interest in playing with same-sex peers, or emulating same-sex fantasy models, and has toy and activity interests more typical of the other gender. **Adolescence** The adolescent is isolated from the same-sex peer group, finds little in common with same-sex peers, is teased for manifesting cross-gender behaviors, expresses occasional regret that he or she was not born as a member of the opposite sex.
	SPECIAL INFORMATION
	For cross-gender problems, as opposed to disorder, the child does not completely reject gender role attributes typical of his or her sex. It is likely, however, that the boundary between problem and disorder is closer than the boundary between problem and developmental variation. It would be rare to diagnose a cross-gender behavior PROBLEM as compared to a developmental VARIATION (e.g., tomboy) or DISORDER (see following section). Any time a parent is concerned about a child's cross-gender activities, the child and his family should be referred for evaluation by a mental health professional who can interpret the significance of the child's behavior in the context of family dynamics.

DISORDER	COMMON DEVELOPMENTAL PRESENTATIONS
302.6 Childhood Gender Identity Disorder **302.85 Adolescent Gender Identity Disorder** The display of a strong and persistent desire to be of the opposite sex and persistent discomfort with his or her sex resulting in such activities as cross-dressing and preoccupation with getting rid of secondary sex characteristics. The disturbance is not concurrent with a physical intersex condition. (see *DSM-IV* Criteria Appendix, p 328)	**Infancy** Not relevant at this age. **Early Childhood** The child engages in persistent and pervasive cross-dressing, cross-gender role play, toy play, and peer play over a period of 3 months, frequently states that he or she would like to become a member of the opposite sex, expresses the desire to have anatomic attributes of the opposite sex, rejects any sex-typical behaviors associated with his or her own sex, is teased by peer groups, expresses overt distress that he or she cannot change sex. In a few cases, the child may actually believe that he or she is a member of the opposite sex, but this is rarely seen after age 4 years. **Middle Childhood** The child engages in persistent and pervasive cross-dressing, cross-gender role play, toy play, and peer play that persists over a period of 3 months, frequently states that he or she would like to become a member of the opposite sex, expresses the desire to have anatomic attributes of the opposite sex, strongly rejects any sex-typical behaviors associated with his or her own sex, is teased by peer groups, expresses overt distress that he or she cannot change sex. **Adolescence** Markedly avoids same-sex peers and sex-typical activities, attempts to "pass" socially as a member of the opposite sex by cross-dressing and changes in hairstyle, and may desire sex-modifying procedures, including hormonal and physical interventions.

SPECIAL INFORMATION
Young girls with gender identity disorder not only insist on wearing clothes of the other sex but will become so upset if required to wear a skirt or dress for a special occasion that they may refuse to attend the event. They will often try to pass as a boy by taking on a gender neutral nickname and by cutting their hair very short. Young boys with gender identity disorder often have a compulsion to cross-dress, often to the exclusion of more ordinary play activities. The persistence of the behavior and accompanied distress represents substantial conflict in gender identity formation. Only a small number of children with gender identity disorders will continue to have symptoms that meet the criteria for gender identity disorder in late adolescence or adulthood. Most children with gender identity disorder display less overt cross-gender behaviors with time, parental intervention, or response from peers. Some children with a history of gender identity disorder may become more aware of an erotic attraction to same-sex individuals. They may require a lot of support in clarifying their sexual orientation and integrating their sexual identity into their self-concept. Some adolescents who are not sure of their sexual orientation also may experience an attraction to same-sex individuals and they, too, may need support in clarifying their sexual orientation. It is important to note that adolescents who are trying to sort out their sexual orientation do not usually have a *gender identity disorder.*

DIFFERENTIAL DIAGNOSIS	SPECIAL INFORMATION
General Medical Conditions Not relevant.	Children with physical intersex conditions rarely have gender identity disorder. In some conditions, children may display more extensive cross-gender behavior than is typical for their genetic sex. For example, girls with congenital adrenal hyperplasia may have increased athletic interests, but rarely have gender identity problems or disorders. In part, this is understood to be a function of the effects of prenatal overexposure to male sex hormones on the developing central nervous system.
Substances Not relevant.	
Mental Disorders Not relevant.	

COMMONLY COMORBID CONDITIONS	SPECIAL INFORMATION
Other Comorbid Mental Health Conditions — Examples include: 309.21 Separation anxiety disorder 300.02 Generalized anxiety disorder 300.4 Dysthymic disorder V40.3 Social withdrawal problem 296.2x, Major depressive disorder 296.3x 309.81 Posttraumatic stress disorder 995.53 Sexual abuse 313.9 Suicidal ideation and attempts	These associated problems in children who are unable to resolve their conflict about gender identity are compounded with age as they become repeatedly stigmatized by peers. It is further compounded by the fact that the disorder occurs most often in families experiencing ongoing stress and where parents have unresolved emotional difficulties. Adolescents with gender identity disorder are frequently depressed (see Sadness and Related Symptoms cluster, p 153), drop out of school, and experience suicidal ideation (see Suicidal Behaviors cluster, p 165). In youths from lower socioeconomic circumstances, prostitution and substance abuse (see Substance Use/Abuse cluster, p 135) are common.
Other General Medical Conditions Not relevant.	

Presenting Complaints

plays with genitals
sexual play with other children
excessive sexual curiosity
masturbation
excessive masturbation
precocious sexual activity
exposing genitals to others

Definitions and Symptoms

The presenting complaints represent widely diverse behaviors that all relate to the developing sexuality of the infant, child, and adolescent. Some of the behaviors involve touching and/or manipulating one's own genitals or those of others. Other behaviors are thought to be associated with sexual arousal or the communication of sexual feelings to others, and yet other behaviors involve sexual identity and/or sexual fantasy.

In infancy and early childhood, exploration of one's own genitals and those of other children is very common. Preschool children are typically very curious about their own sexual organs and those of other children and adults. Masturbation at this age is frequently seen, though less commonly than sexual exploration or play. An increase in all these behaviors is noted with higher levels of arousal and in situations of isolation or neglect when the self-stimulating effects of the behaviors may be sought. During early school age years, sexual feelings are universal but expression is typically suppressed by social convention. Sexual behaviors at this age typically occur in private or in small groups of same-sex peers. During adolescence, there is a sharp increase in sexual arousal that is hormonally produced and expressions of sexuality increase dramatically, although they are highly modified by cultural and religious expectations. Sexual behavior of varying degrees is expected and accepted in relationships with others. Masturbation is extremely common. During school age and adolescence, problem degrees of sexual behaviors are strongly related to level of maturity, degree of impulsivity, the impact of harmful experiences such as abuse, and the expectations of family and peers.

In infancy and early childhood, these behaviors are typically reported by the caregiver on the basis of their observations. Caregivers frequently seek advice on how to manage these behaviors even though the behaviors themselves are within normal limits, because expressions of sexuality frequently arouse anxiety in adults.

Epidemiology

Some degree of sexual arousal and/or sexual curiosity is a universal part of human experience. However, the definition of what constitutes a sexual problem is so extensively influenced by psychological, cultural, and religious bias that there is little agreement on the incidence of most of these behaviors.

Etiology

Sexual behaviors have their origin primarily as expressions of the arousal of sexual feelings and/or in exploration based upon curiosity. Therefore, the extent and intensity of the behaviors relate to the degree of sexual arousal experienced and the person's level of curiosity. The expression of these feelings is powerfully modified by parental response and religious and cultural expectations.

DEVELOPMENTAL VARIATION	COMMON DEVELOPMENTAL PRESENTATIONS
V65.49 Sexual Behaviors Variation Sexual behaviors that reflect pleasure in genital stimulation and/or curiosity about one's own or other people's genitals are expected behaviors across the developmental range. The open expression of these behaviors is expected in infancy and early childhood but normally becomes private as universal cultural taboos restrict the open expression of sexuality, especially with others.	**Infancy** Touching genitals; erections in infant boys. **Early Childhood** The child touches and explores own genitals; curiosity includes touching and exploring genitals of other children; masturbation, occasionally, but *not* compulsively; use of bathroom language in jokes and teasing; sexually provocative behavior towards adults of opposite gender, especially parents of opposite gender. **Middle Childhood** The child explores his or her own genitals in private; curiosity is manifested by looking at sexual books or magazines; the child masturbates in private; mutual sex play occasionally occurs in same-sex consenting groups. **Adolescence** The adolescent masturbates in private or in same-sex consensual groups; curiosity is manifested by perusal of sexual books, magazines, or videos; consensual nonintercourse sexual contact (e.g., "petting") occurs with opposite or same-sex partners.

SPECIAL INFORMATION
These normal expressions of sexuality are often a problem for caregivers based on their own level of comfort with normal sexual expression. There are wide variations in cultural and religious beliefs that may affect caregiver attitudes. The expression of sexuality is closely related to caregiver reactions along with the degree to which the child is compliant or oppositional. The expression of sexuality in adolescents is powerfully affected by the peer group, which, in turn, is responsive to community cultural norms. These factors must be understood in order to evaluate the degree of pathology associated with some behaviors. Adolescents who are gay or lesbian may first acknowledge their sexual orientation in mid or late adolescence. It is important that physicians who care for teenagers be prepared to recognize and acknowledge an adolescent's homosexual orientation.

PROBLEM	COMMON DEVELOPMENTAL PRESENTATIONS
V40.3 Sexual Behaviors Problem These behaviors become a problem when: 1) the behavior has a compulsive quality and occurs more often than other normal childhood behaviors; 2) the behaviors have begun to mimic the sexual behaviors of older individuals, suggesting inappropriate stimulation by older people; and/or 3) the behaviors begin to violate cultural norms of privacy and/or violate the individual rights of others. However, the behaviors remain a problem as long as the above characteristics are not sufficiently intense to qualify for the diagnosis of sexual disorder, NOS.	**Infancy** Not usually relevant at this age. **Early Childhood** Masturbation is frequent and may interfere with other, normal activities; curiosity is excessive but not obsessional; the child is occasionally provocative in sexual teasing. **Middle Childhood** Masturbation is occasionally open, rather than private; the child seems occasionally preoccupied with sexual books or magazines; the child engages in sexual play with another child occasionally. **Adolescence** Masturbation or perusal of sexual books and magazines is excessive and occasionally interrupts other age-appropriate activities; non-intercourse sexual contact occurs earlier than is usually anticipated; sexual intercourse may occur earlier than is normal for the peer and cultural group.
	SPECIAL INFORMATION
	In early childhood the degree of stimulation produced by inappropriate exposure to adult sexuality must be considered (see p 00). This includes a history of sexual abuse. The child who is immature and/or impulsive is more likely to engage in sexual behaviors inappropriately.

DISORDER	COMMON DEVELOPMENTAL PRESENTATIONS
302.9 Sexual Disorder, Not Otherwise Specified This *DSM-IV* classification includes specific disorders such as paraphilias, but these are usually not relevant for most children. This nonspecific diagnosis can be used when problematic behaviors are severe. This should include the situations where the behaviors are compulsive, considerably advanced for the child's developmental age, and violate cultural norms of privacy and the rights of others.	**Infancy** Not usually relevant at this age. **Early Childhood** Repetitive and self-absorbed masturbation. Play themes involve adult-level sexual behavior. **Middle Childhood** Masturbation and genital manipulation is compulsive and lacks awareness of privacy. Repeated attempts are made to engage others in sexual play or masturbation, particularly younger playmates. **Adolescence** The adolescent engages in promiscuous or indiscriminate sexual behavior including developmentally early and excessive sexual intercourse and multiple partners. Sexual aggressiveness may occur, including rape or other forced sexual activity. Voyeurism is repeated and compulsive in quality. Masturbation or other sexual activity occurs without regard to privacy.
	SPECIAL INFORMATION
	Sexually indiscriminate behavior may result from sexual abuse (see p 45), and this possibility should always be considered. Girls with attention-deficit/hyperactivity disorders and conduct problems disorder are at risk to act out sexually in adolescence (see Hyperactive/Impulsive Behaviors cluster, p 93, and Inattention Behaviors cluster, p 103).

DIFFERENTIAL DIAGNOSIS	SPECIAL INFORMATION
General Medical Conditions Endocrine disorders may result in precocious sexual development. Examples include: Precocious puberty Adreno-genital syndrome, especially in females XYY male	Code the endocrine disorder only if correction of the endocrine disorder alleviates the behaviors (otherwise code both conditions). In the absence of any other significant psychopathology, the sexual behavior is in keeping with the sexual, rather than chronological, age. Females with sexual precocity may have problems with inappropriate sexually provocative behavior.
Substances Substance use is associated with a loss or reduction of inhibition and, especially in adolescents, often results in inappropriate sexual behavior, including behaviors that intrude on the rights of others.	Code the substance use and the sexual problem or disorder.
Mental Disorders Severe mental disorders such as schizophrenia or bipolar disorder may result in loss of inhibitions with sexual acting out.	Code the mental disorder only.

COMMONLY COMORBID CONDITIONS	SPECIAL INFORMATION
Other Comorbid Mental Health Conditions — Examples include: 300.02 Generalized anxiety disorder 300.3 Obsessive-compulsive disorder 312.81 Conduct disorder childhood onset 312.82 Conduct disorder adolescent onset (particularly when associated with ADHD) 296.2x, Major depressive disorder 296.3x 300.4 Dysthymia 313.9 Suicidal ideation and attempts 309.xx Adjustment disorder 305.xx Substance abuse disorder	These chronic behavioral disorders often include the behaviors of immaturity, poor social judgment, and impulsivity that contribute to sexual behavior problems and/or disorders. Code both conditions. Disorders involving depressed mood may result in sexual acting out, especially during adolescence. The sexual behaviors are often pursued in an attempt to compensate for low self-esteem. Code both conditions.
Other General Medical Conditions Any chronic medical condition that significantly impairs self-esteem may result in compensatory sexual acting out, especially in adolescence. Examples include: Cystic fibrosis Sickle cell disease Diabetes mellitus	

Atypical Behaviors

Repetitive Behavioral Patterns

Social Interaction Behaviors

Bizarre Behaviors

Presenting Complaints

thumb sucking

head banging

hair pulling

tics

rocking

hand flaps

slaps/bites self

Definitions and Symptoms

Repetitive behaviors are common, often rhythmical patterns of behaviors that occur repeatedly. They appear to serve no socially acceptable purpose, although they may serve to comfort the child. These behaviors, although common in normally developing children, are frequently seen in association with delayed or atypical development. Certain patterns of repetitive behaviors, in particular self-injurious behaviors, may indicate an underlying pathology or disorder (Lesch-Nyhan syndrome) and should not be viewed as merely a normal variation. Repetitive behaviors include thumb sucking, head banging, hair pulling, tics, and pica. Thumb sucking is typically associated with sleep or stressful situations and may be momentary or last for hours. Finger sucking, blanket sucking, and tongue sucking are related phenomena. In head banging, on awakening or at bedtime, the child repeatedly strikes his or her head against a solid object, often the crib. The child may be on his or her hands and knees, sitting, or prone. The repetition typically lasts 15 minutes but may go on for hours. Despite seeming discomfort, the child does not appear to experience pain. Hair pulling may range from gentle repetitive traction on the hair to pulling out, rubbing off, and twisting out hair or cutting it with a pair of scissors. The hair involved may be on the scalp, eyebrows, eyelashes, or pubic area. Hair pulling may result in areas of alopecia. Tics are involuntary, sudden, rapid, recurrent, nonrhythmic stereotyped motor movements or vocalizations that typically mimic some aspect of normal behavior such as eye blink or cough. Examples of *motor tics* include eye blinking, facial grimacing, neck stretching, sniffing, or repeated swallowing. Examples of *vocal tics* include grunts, barks, yelps, throat clearing, coughing, echolalia, and coprolalia. The disorders include transient tic disorder (motor or vocal tics that are present for at least 4 weeks but less than 12 consecutive months), chronic motor or vocal tic disorder (lasting longer than 1 year but involving only motor or vocal tics but not both), and Tourette's disorder (the presence of both motor and vocal tics during some part of the illness, variation in the pattern of tics over time, and occurring multiple times daily or intermittently for at least 1 year). *Pica* is the persistent ingestion of nonfood substances such as dirt, hair, paint, animal droppings, or pebbles. The onset of these behaviors may follow a stressful environmental event (see Environmental Situations Defined, p 31). In nonverbal individuals with severe mental retardation, the behaviors may be triggered by a painful general medical condition, boredom, or the desire to avoid situations.

Epidemiology

Estimates of the prevalence of self-injurious behaviors in individuals with mental retardation vary from 2% to 3% in children and adolescents living in the community to approximately 25% in adults with severe or profound mental retardation living in institutions (see Cognitive Adaptive Skills cluster, p 61).

DEVELOPMENTAL VARIATION	COMMON DEVELOPMENTAL PRESENTATIONS
V65.49 Repetitive Behaviors Variation Sporadic repetitive movements such as rocking, head banging, or hair twisting that are of limited duration, cause no physical harm, and do not impair normal development or activities.	**Infancy** The infant rocks in the crib when seated or on his or her hands and knees, sucks thumb, exhibits head banging, twists hair, and exhibits pica. These behaviors increase with hunger and fatigue. **Early Childhood** The child rocks when seated watching television, when not otherwise occupied, or when anxious, usually in small movements, and has head and shoulder movements often accompanied by mouthing fingers or thumb sucking, head banging, hair pulling, eye blinking, or pica. **Middle Childhood** The child twirls or twists hair, pulls at ear lobes, repeatedly picks nose, repeatedly rubs eyes, and exhibits occasional tics. **Adolescence** Repetitive behaviors seldom occur in adolescence, although hair twirling or twisting and similar nonfunctional "picking" at body parts occurs.
	SPECIAL INFORMATION
	Thumb sucking is extremely common in children under 4 years (45%) and decreases in frequency thereafter. Head banging disappears in most children by age 4 years but may persist. Early onset hair pulling (before 6 years) tends to be self-limited, whereas later onset tends to be more severe and long lasting. Normal rocking and thumb sucking are distinguished by their relative ease of interruption. Picking behaviors may continue, especially when the youth is anxious (see Anxious Symptoms cluster, p 145). All of these behaviors increase in situations of anxiety or boredom.

PROBLEM	COMMON DEVELOPMENTAL PRESENTATIONS
V40.3 Repetitive Behaviors Problem Repetitive behaviors can cause some social disruption and/or dysfunction that results from the behavior itself and from the responses of others to that behavior but is not sufficiently intense to qualify for a diagnosis of the repetitive behaviors disorder.	**Infancy** The infant rocks in his or her crib causing bruises or callouses, waves hands and arms, which occasionally slap the face, and bites into thumb when sucking, causing lesions. **Early Childhood** The child rocks for long periods of time when alone, with large movements from the waist, but can be interrupted when spoken to or when a distracting sound occurs, inserts objects into ears and nostrils, and persistently sucks thumb after age 4 years, especially in public. **Middle Childhood** The child picks and pulls at skin or nails causing small scratches and bleeding, repeatedly picks nose causing nosebleeds, inserts pencils, pins, or other objects into the ear canals and/or nostrils causing bleeding and infections, and pulls hair, producing some hair loss that becomes socially stigmatizing. **Adolescence** The adolescent produces excoriation of skin associated with acne, but this persists after the acute lesions have healed, bites fingernails until they bleed or may become infected, and pulls hair that begins to be socially stigmatizing.
	SPECIAL INFORMATION
	Although these behaviors are extremely common, their persistence may lead to humiliation, social rejection, academic dysfunction, and other difficulties. Pica may lead to poisoning from paint chip ingestion or toxoplasmosis. Head banging may frequently result in contusion and callous formation, whereas brain damage and retinal detachment are rare.

DISORDER	COMMON DEVELOPMENTAL PRESENTATIONS
There are a group of disorders that entail repetitive movements but are not necessarily related in their manifestations or in who presents with them. Stereotypic movement disorder most commonly presents in children with mental retardation. The developmental presentations refer to stereotypic movement disorder. The other disorders have less changes that occur in the course of development. **307.3 Stereotypic Movement Disorder** The essential feature is motor behavior that is repetitive, often seemingly driven, and nonfunctional. At this level, the behaviors are clearly associated with social dysfunction and stigmatization. (see *DSM-IV* Criteria Appendix, p 347) **312.39 Trichotillomania** Recurrent pulling out of one's hair resulting in noticeable hair loss. Stressful situations frequently increase hair pulling behavior. For some, an increasing sense of tension occurs immediately before pulling out the hair or when attempting to resist the behavior. The individual experiences pleasure, gratification, or relief when pulling out the hair. (see *DSM-IV* Criteria Appendix, p 350) **307.21 Transient Tic Disorder** Single or multiple motor and/or vocal tics that occur many times a day, nearly every day for at least 4 weeks but for no longer than 12 consecutive months. **307.22 Chronic Motor or Vocal Tic Disorder** Single or multiple motor or vocal tics, but not both, have been present at some time during the illness. The tics occur many times a day nearly every day or intermittently throughout a period of more than 1 year. The disturbance causes marked distress or significant impairment in social or academic functioning. **307.23 Tourette's Disorder** Both multiple motor and one or more vocal tics have been present at some time during the illness. The tics occur many times a day nearly every day or intermittently throughout a period of more than 1 year.	**Infancy** The infant slaps his or her face, engages in head banging on the crib while rocking, causing bruising, and has repetitive movements that are difficult to interrupt, causing screaming, flailing arms, and kicking. **Early Childhood** The child hits his or her face or ears with fists, inserts fingers up into nostrils or ear canals causing lesions and bleeding, severely rocks accompanied by periodic bouts of banging the head or limbs against hard objects or surfaces, kicks against hard objects with bare feet, shins, or knees, and strikes the chest or abdomen with fists. The child repeatedly pulls out his or her hair and/or engages in multiple motor tics and one or more vocal tics. **Middle Childhood** The child repeatedly hits self or head against hard objects and bites self, including the wrists, hands, and forearms. The child repeatedly pulls out his or her hair and/or engages in multiple motor tics and one or more vocal tics. **Adolescence** The adolescent exhibits severe head banging or self-biting. The adolescent repeatedly pulls out one's hair and/or performs multiple motor and one or more vocal tics. **SPECIAL INFORMATION** Repetitive behaviors that result in frequent self-injury should be referred to a mental health clinician. For stereotypic movement disorder, head slapping or hitting may persist for minutes at a time so severely that the child bleeds. Self-biting causes lesions and deep indentations in skin. Banging behavior is very persistent and very difficult to interrupt (usually verbal interruption does not stop the behavior for more than a few seconds or minutes). For stereotypic movement disorder in adolescence, severe banging or self-biting may last for several minutes a bout, and overall may last hours with interpolated rest periods if not interrupted. The behavior invariably causes some form of contusions, lesions, or sores. If the youth is restrained, he or she will struggle against the restraints to become free to resume self-injury. The youth, when not engaging in self-injuring behavior, will actively hand flap and make screaming or screeching sounds when excited. For stereotypic movement disorder, children who look "glassy-eyed" as they rock or face slap and are difficult to distract are more likely to have a serious developmental disorder; distinguish intermittent self-inflicted injuries in peripheral neuropathy from stereotypic self-injury. Stereotypic movement disorder may be specified with self-injurious behavior if the behavior results in bodily change that requires specific treatment.

DIFFERENTIAL DIAGNOSIS	SPECIAL INFORMATION
General Medical Conditions — Examples include: Multiple sclerosis Postviral encephalitis Head injury *Stereotypic movement disorder:* Deafness Blindness Peripheral neuropathy Otitis media Cornelia deLange syndrome Fragile X syndrome Teething *Trichotillomania:* Alopecia areata Tinea capitis Ringworm Pyoderma *Transient tic disorder:* Sydenham chorea Huntington's chorea Choreoathetosis Hemiballismus	Movement and seizure disorder may mimic tics. Allergic symptoms can mimic throat clearing and sniffing. Self-stimulating behaviors in individuals with sensory deficits (blindness, deafness) usually do not result in dysfunction or self-injury.
Substances — Examples include: Seizure medications Antithyroid *Stereotypic movement disorder:* Sedatives Hypnotic, anxiolytic, benzodiazepine *Trichotillomania:* Cytotoxic Anticoagulant *Transient tic disorder:* Excessive caffeinated beverages Amphetamines Methylphenidate	Self-injury behaviors can be exacerbated when sedative, hypnotic, anxiolytic, and/or benzodiazepines or seizure medications are administered to people with mental retardation who are prone to self-injury. High doses of stimulant medication can cause self-"picking" behavior at cuticles or scabs; stimulant and antidepressant medication can exacerbate tics.
Mental Disorders Stereotypic movement disorder: **299.00** Autistic disorder and other pervasive developmental disorders	Tourette's disorder typically occurs between 2 and 15 years of age, with a median age of 7 years. Stereotypic movement disorder can be diagnosed in the presence of mental retardation, if the behavior is severe enough to be a focus of treatment, but do not diagnose stereotypic movement disorder if the symptoms are part of a pervasive developmental disorder or trichotillomania.

COMMONLY COMORBID CONDITIONS	SPECIAL INFORMATION
Other Comorbid Mental Health Conditions — Examples include: *Stereotypic movement disorder:* **317,** Mental retardation **318.x,** **319** *Transient tic disorder:* **313.81** Oppositional defiant disorder **312.81** Conduct disorder childhood onset **312.82** Conduct disorder adolescent onset **312.9** Disruptive behavior disorder not otherwise specified **300.3** Obsessive-compulsive disorder **314.xx** Attention-deficit/hyperactivity disorder	Stereotypic movements may be associated with mental retardation, especially for individuals in nonstimulating environments. Repetitive stereotyped movements are a characteristic feature of pervasive developmental disorders, and no separate diagnosis is made. Self-mutilation, especially cutting and burning, occurs in children who have been abused (see p 45).
Other General Medical Conditions — Examples include: Malocclusion Cerebral contusion/concussion Retinal hemorrhage Lead intoxication Intestinal obstruction secondary to trichobezoar Infections secondary to ingestion of fecal material Chronic tissue damage (bruises, bite marks, scratches) Chronic skin irritation or calluses from biting, pinching, scratching, or saliva smearing *Stereotypic movement disorder:* Lesch-Nyhan syndrome Prader-Willi syndrome	

Presenting Complaints

qualitative impairments in reciprocal social interaction and
 communication (and restricted, repetitive, and
 stereotyped patterns of behavior, interests, and activities)

rarely plays or interacts with other children (especially in
 group situations)

has no (few) friends

does not speak

has stopped speaking

often does not appear to hear or listen to what others say

has trouble conversing with others

does not pay attention

is hyperactive

has no sense of danger

is negative and stubborn

gets upset and has tantrums easily

often behaves in an embarrassing manner

insistence on routines and rituals

stereotypic movements

Definitions and Symptoms

From the early neonatal period onward, infants and children are highly social beings. They appear to be "pre-wired" for social interaction, preferentially attending and responding (in reciprocal fashion) to social stimuli. Very young infants recognize and respond differentially to their caregivers by using sensory information. During the first months of life, reciprocal social interactions develop, including responsive smiling and reciprocal eye gaze, facial expressions, and vocalizations. Between the ages of 6 months and 3 years, a variety of social behaviors develop, including attachment behaviors, stranger recognition, social imitation and mimicry, joint attention (the mutual sharing of observations and interests), separation distress, curiosity about new adults and children, and pretend play. In addition, social communication develops and includes speech and a variety of nonverbal forms of communication (e.g., pointing and reciprocal eye contact, directed facial and vocal expressions and gestures such as waving or signaling others to come near or sit beside them).

Infants and young children are typically interested in a wide variety of activities and approach novel situations with curiosity and exploratory behavior (possibly with some initial anxiety). They develop the capacity for functional and symbolic toy and object use and later become capable of deductive, hypothetical reasoning and problem solving.

Older children develop an appreciation for social rules and expectations (which are often subtle) and are usually motivated to please caregivers, teachers, and others by adhering to these expectations. They develop an increasing interest in playing cooperatively with other children, developing friendships, and sharing interests, confidences, and personal issues with their peers. Participation in social group activities and becoming a member of a social group are increasingly important.

Although there are normal variations in the acquisition and expression of these social and communicative aspects of development, interest in others and the capacity to relate in a reciprocal manner are innate.

Autism and other pervasive development disorders (PDDs) involve fundamental deficits in social reciprocity (e.g., joint attention, shared experience, social cognition), pragmatic communication (conversation, "chat," social gesture), and in the range and breadth of preferred interests and activities. Atypical and dramatic responses to change, unusual sensory interests, and stereotypic patterns of behavior are also common in these syndromes. Other features related to autism include compulsions, which are repetitive and seemingly purposeful behaviors enacted according to certain rules or in a stereotyped fashion, and uneven skill development, in which very rare cases are savant skills (areas of significant talent that exceed the overall abilities of the individual and of the general population). The accurate diagnosis of autistic disorder and the other PDDs may lead to appropriate medical assessments and in early interventions which may improve the long-term prognosis.

Epidemiology

Epidemiologic data suggest that 4 to 13 children in 10,000 fit within the Autistic-PDD Spectrum.

Etiology

Autism and related PDDs are early onset conditions of neurobiological origin. In some instances, the etiology can be determined (e.g., congenital rubella, tuberous sclerosis, fragile X syndrome); in the majority of cases, however, the specific etiology remains elusive.

DEVELOPMENTAL VARIATION	COMMON DEVELOPMENTAL PRESENTATIONS
V65.49 Social Interaction Variation Because of constitutional and/or psychological factors, children and adolescents will vary in their ability and desire to interact with other people. Less socially adept or desirous children do not have a problem as long as it does not interfere with their normal development and activities.	**Infancy** Infants exhibit a variety of individual differences in terms of reactivity to sensation (underreactive or overreactive), capacity to process information in auditory, visual modes, as well as motor tone, motor planning, and movement patterns. For example, some babies are underreactive to touch and sound, with low motor tone, and may appear self-absorbed and require a great deal of parental wooing and engagement to be responsive. The ease with which the caregivers can mobilize a baby by dealing with the infant's individually different pattern suggests a variation rather than a problem or disorder. **Early Childhood** The child is self-absorbed, enjoys solitary play, with and without fantasy, but can be wooed into relating and interacting by a caregiver who tailors his or her response to individual differences. The child may be slightly slower in his or her language development and not make friends easily. **Middle Childhood** The child may not make friends easily and be less socially adept. The child may prefer solitary play at times. **Adolescence** The adolescent has limited concern regarding popular dress, interests, and activities. The adolescent finds it difficult to make friends at times.
	SPECIAL INFORMATION
	Consider expressive language disorder or mixed receptive-expressive language disorder.

PROBLEM	COMMON DEVELOPMENTAL PRESENTATIONS
V40.3 Social Withdrawal Problem The child's inability and/or desire to interact with people is limited enough to begin to interfere with the child's development and activities.	**Infancy** The infant has an unusually high threshold and/or low intensity of response, is irritable, difficult to console, overly complacent, may exhibit head banging or other repetitive behavior. The infant requires persistent wooing and engagement, including, at times, highly pleasurable and challenging sensory and affective experiences, to keep from remaining self-absorbed and withdrawing. **Early Childhood** The child shows self-absorption, and prefers solitary play. The child has some verbal and/or nonverbal communication, is mildly compulsive, and shows rigid behaviors. **Middle Childhood** The child is very shy, reticent, shows an increased concern about order and rules, is socially isolated, rarely initiates peer interactions, and prefers solitary activities to peer group activities. **Adolescence** The adolescent shows difficulty in social situations, has limited friendships, is socially isolated, may be a "loner," prefers solitary activities to peer group activities, is reticent, has eccentric hobbies and interests, and has limited concern regarding popular styles of dress, behavior, or role models.
	SPECIAL INFORMATION
	Consider sensory impairments (vision, hearing). Excessive sensory stimulation may increase anxiety and agitation. There are children with initial symptoms severe enough to be considered as having an autistic disorder, who with appropriate and full intervention, will markedly improve.

DISORDER	COMMON DEVELOPMENTAL PRESENTATIONS
299.00 Autistic Disorder **Spectrum Pervasive Developmental Disorders** Children diagnosed in the PDD category evidence a wide range of clinical features and developmental capacities. At the more competent level are children who evidence intermittent capacities for warmth and reciprocity but in a highly immature way. They also show delayed communication but have some intentional use of words, gestures, and may evidence some beginning pretend play. These children also often evidence underlying processing difficulties that can appear as irregular motor and sensory patterns. At the lower end of this range are children who may closely fit the description of classic autism. While these children evidence severe patterns of avoidance and lack of symbolic capacities, many still evidence fleeting capacities for gestural and simple communication, warmth and relatedness with trusted caregivers. Autistic disorder is the prototype and will be discussed in this section. The core clinical features of autism and related PDDs constitute a triad of behavioral characteristics in social interactions, verbal and nonverbal communication, and repetitive activities and interests. These features include qualitative impairments in social, communicative, and behavioral aspects of development. The social difficulties involve deficits in the ability to form reciprocal, give-and-take relationships, express empathy, process social cues appropriately, and develop friendships. Great difficulty is encountered in understanding the rules and expectations that govern social interaction and discourse. Significant deficits are present in the pragmatic (social) aspects of both verbal and nonverbal communication. Speech may be limited or absent. When present, it is often overly formal, pedantic, perseverative, idiosyncratic, and/or echolalic. Speech prosody (intonation, inflection, cadence) is atypical. Nonverbal communication is also impaired, with limited use and understanding of reciprocal eye contact, facial expressions, vocal intonation, and social gestures. The behavioral profile includes circumscribed interests, marked distress in response to change, stereotypic mannerisms, and unusual preoccupations, sensory interests, and attachments to objects.	**Infancy** The infant has significant limitations in social smiling, reciprocal eye contact, vocalization with caregivers, social imitative play (peek-a-boo, pat-a-cake), and speech and social gestures. Some young infants may only manifest very subtle differences in social responsivity (the need to work to keep the baby engaged) and evidence the more obvious and negative social withdrawal and/or a regression in existing communicative capacities somewhere between 16 and 24 months. By the second year of life, some infants may exhibit sensory underreactivity or overreactivity, auditory and visual-spatial processing, reduced muscle tone, and motor planning difficulties. While some infants are described as irritable, some are actually described as easy infants. **Early Childhood** The child has difficulty communicating desires for closeness and comfort and may appear isolated and aloof. The child has difficulty with give-and-take behavior, has restricted range of facial and vocal expressions, has limited social gestures, has little curiosity or interest in playing and interacting with other children, often does not respond to the questions and comments of others, displays echolalia (parroting the statements of others), has limited pretend play, engages in repetitive motor behavior (flapping arms, toe-walking), has attachments to unusual objects (rubber bands, sticks), engages in repetitive use of objects, becomes markedly anxious and agitated in response to minor changes in routine or environment, has impaired social communication, has unusual and restricted interests, and speech is delayed or absent. Evidence of sensory underactivity or overactivity, auditory and visual-spatial processing, reduced muscle tone, and motor planning difficulties may be found. **Middle Childhood** The child rarely offers comfort to others, rarely shares pleasure and excitement with others, is aloof, has restricted social and vocal expressiveness, has limited social gestures, has few or no friends, has limited understanding or interest in group games and activities, rarely plays imaginatively with other children, has limited reciprocal conversation, displays echolalia, displays perseverative speech, has unusual speech tone and rhythm, becomes markedly anxious and agitated in response to minor changes in routine or environment, engages in compulsive, ritualistic behaviors, displays motor stereotypy, and has unusual interests. **Adolescence** The adolescent has deficits in the understanding of social rules and expectations, displays unusual expressions of affect (laughs inappropriately), has limited friendships, engages in limited reciprocal conversations, perseverates, displays echolalic speech, is ritualistic, and has compulsive behaviors (see Ritualistic, Obsessive, Compulsive Symptoms cluster, p 161). Adolescents with this disorder can become aggressive and a challenge to manage.

DISORDER, CONTINUED	SPECIAL INFORMATION
The expression of the symptoms outlined will vary greatly from child to child. Diagnosis is established by the pattern of symptoms as they relate to the triad of behavioral characteristics. The following disorders are included: autistic disorder, Rett's disorder, childhood disintegrative disorder, Asperger's disorder, and PDD not otherwise specified (NOS). Currently a wide range of developmental patterns are diagnosed in the PDD-NOS category. There is a difference of opinion about whether these disorders represent a qualitatively distinct neurobiological disease characterized by a primary deficit in both relating and communicating, or whether the clinical features of this disorder are a secondary reaction to an underlying series of processing and modulation deficits in the areas of auditory, visual-spatial, motor, and other sensory processing patterns. They all have impairments in social interaction and communication. In children with Asperger's disorder, language and cognitive are not significantly delayed, whereas in children with autistic disorder they are frequently delayed. With Rhett's and childhood disintegrative disorders the symptoms are more severe and progressive. This developmental profile results in significant distress and/or functional impairment. (see *DSM-IV* Criteria Appendix, p 311) **299.00** Autistic disorder (see p 316) **299.80** Rett's disorder (see p 341) **299.80** Asperger's disorder (see p 315) **299.10** Childhood disintegrative disorder (see p 321) **299.80** PDD, NOS	See *DSM-IV* Criteria Appendix, p 311. Development is considered qualitatively atypical, not simply delayed. If a PDD is suspected, refer the patient for a comprehensive evaluation. If the child has a PDD, do not diagnose ADHD (see Hyperactive/Impulsive Behaviors cluster, p 93, and Inattentive Behaviors cluster, p 103). The developmental abnormality must be manifest by delays or abnormal functioning in at least one of the following areas prior to 3 years of age: social interaction, language as used in social communication, or symbolic or imaginative play. Rates of the disorder are four to five times higher in males than in females. However, females with the disorder are more likely to exhibit more severe mental retardation. The stress of having a child with autism can have secondary effects on marital and family functioning. The individuals with autism are at higher risk for developing a seizure disorder. Many children experience severe processing deficits in terms of auditory, visual-spatial, and motor planning patterns, as well as reacting to sensation.

DIFFERENTIAL DIAGNOSIS	SPECIAL INFORMATION

General Medical Conditions —
Examples include:
Developmental or acquired aphasia
   (Landau-Kleffner syndrome)
Congenital infections (congenital rubella)
Metabolic disorders (phenylketonuria)
Genetic disorders (fragile X syndrome,
   tuberous sclerosis)
Encephalitis
Anoxia during birth
Maternal rubella
	These conditions, with the exception of Landau-Kleffner syndrome, sometimes but not always appear to cause symptoms warranting the diagnosis of autism or other PDDs. Different than most other conditions, both conditions are diagnosed since the general medical condition does not necessarily imply the PDD condition even though it may be causal in autism and other PDDs more often than would be anticipated on the basis of developmental level alone.
	
	Even though the medical condition may cause the disorder, since many children with the medical condition do not have that disorder, code both if present.

Substances — Examples include: Lead poisoning Amphetamines Methylphenidate	These substances can cause behavioral symptoms (hyperactivity, social withdrawal, stereotypy) that may be erroneously attributed to a PDD. Lead poisoning may cause the symptoms on a permanent basis and should be considered as the general medical condition.

Mental Disorders
300.23 Social phobia
309.21 Separation anxiety disorder
313.23 Selective mutism
313.81 Oppositional deviant disorder
300.3 Obsessive-compulsive disorder
295.xx Schizophrenia, childhood onset
301.20 Schizoid personality disorder
301.22 Schizotypal personality disorder
315.31 Mixed receptive-expressive
   language disorder
299.80 Rett's disorder
299.10 Childhood disintegrative disorder
299.80 Asperger's disorder
317, Mental retardation
318.x,
319
307.3 Stereotypic movement disorder
314.xx Attention-deficit/hyperactivity
   disorder (ADHD)
	A diagnosis of PDD preempts the following: obsessive-compulsive disorder, avoidant disorder, reactive attachment disorder, specific speech and language disorders, and ADHD.
	
	A diagnosis of schizophrenia can be made if an individual with autism develops active phase symptoms of schizophrenia. Childhood-onset schizophrenia is an extremely rare condition that includes a withdrawal from previously established relationships, atypical thought processes (tangential, loosely associated speech), delusional thinking, and altered perceptual experiences (hallucinations, illusions). Adult criteria for schizophrenia are applicable to children and adolescents (see *DSM-IV* Criteria Appendix, p 311). It is also possible, however, for someone with a preexisting PDD to develop schizophrenia at some point later in life (typically during adolescence or young adulthood).

COMMONLY COMORBID CONDITIONS	SPECIAL INFORMATION
Other Comorbid Mental Health Conditions — Examples include: **317,** Mental retardation **318.x,** **319**	Mental retardation is present in approximately 75% of children with autistic disorder, commonly in the moderate range (IQ 35 to 50).
Other General Medical Conditions — Examples include: Seizure disorders Tuberous sclerosis Self-injurious behavior Other conditions secondary to the causative medical condition	Seizure disorders occur in 25% of cases (often with onset during adolescence). Electroencephalographic abnormalities are common even in the absence of seizure disorders.

Presenting Complaints

agitation
cognitive impairment
confusion
disorientation
fluctuation or impairment in level of consciousness
fluctuation in ability to maintain attention
lethargy
memory impairment

Definitions and Symptoms

Delirium is an important clue to the presence of an underlying physical disorder or substance intoxication and should alert the clinician to the likelihood of an unstable or serious medical condition. In the past, such patients were commonly referred to as encephalopathic. The essential feature of delirium is an impairment in consciousness or arousal; fluctuation in the patient's level of consciousness may be evidenced by drowsiness or changes in the sleep-wake cycle. There may be marked changes in activity level, such as the development of lethargy or agitation. Other common findings include a reduced ability to maintain or shift attention, disorientation, disorganized thinking, and memory impairment, particularly disturbance of short-term memory. Sensory input may be distorted or misinterpreted, and perceptual disturbances such as illusions or frank hallucinations may be present. Isolated visual hallucinations are a strong clue to the presence of an undiagnosed physical disorder. Emotional disturbance is common, with patients sometimes appearing irritable, fearful, depressed, or apathetic. Delirium is frequently underdiagnosed, particularly in younger children, where it may be dismissed as "naughty" behavior or as an understandable response to stress. Symptoms tend to fluctuate over the course of the day, often being worse at night. Patients may be dangerous to themselves or others and require close supervision. Substance use or medication side effects can also cause a delirium and in many cases, a combination of a general medical condition and a medication being used to treat that condition both contribute to the delirium.

Psychosis is a more general term, referring to an impairment in reality testing that results from distortions of perception, thinking, or consciousness and is often accompanied by bizarre behavior. Such patients may manifest hallucinations and/or delusions on examination. Delirium may be considered a subcategory of psychosis in the general sense, being distinguished by impairments in arousal and fluctuations in level of consciousness; it serves as an important clue to the presence of physical disease or substance abuse. So-called "functional" psychiatric disorders such as schizophrenia or bipolar disorder are commonly associated with psychosis, but may rarely result in a symptom complex consistent with delirium. The presence of delirium should provoke a careful search for etiologic physical disease or substance use. Dementia is an acquired global impairment of intellect, memory, and personality that occurs without impairment of consciousness; an underlying physical etiology is assumed. Unlike delirium, dementia is rare in children and adolescents, but it does occur as a result of a variety of conditions, including inherited neurodegenerative disorders, toxin exposure, or infections such as human immunodeficiency virus infection. In general, dementia is distinguished from delirium by the relative preservation of consciousness and arousal, as well as a course that is chronic as compared with the more acute course that is more characteristic of delirium.

The clinician may evaluate a child or adolescent who has been identified as behaving in a bizarre or unusual fashion compared with his or her baseline behavior. This may take the form of agitation, withdrawal, or peculiar behaviors. The seriousness of such presentations may range from being relatively benign to emergent, with a change in behavior sometimes signaling the presence of a life-threatening physical condition. For the clinician, it is most important first to determine whether the unusual behavior is the result of a previously undiagnosed or unappreciated physical condition. Certain characteristics of the presentation may help in such an assessment.

Epidemiology

There has been little formal research on delirium in children and adolescents. Children may be more susceptible to delirium than adults, especially when it is related to febrile illness and certain medications (e.g., anticholinergics).

Etiology

Delirium may be produced by virtually any serious medical illness that is significantly advanced and is an indication for a careful medical workup. In equivocal cases, an electroencephalogram may assist in diagnosis by revealing generalized slowing as compared with the patient's baseline.

DEVELOPMENTAL VARIATION	COMMON DEVELOPMENTAL PRESENTATIONS
293.0 Delirium Due To a General Medical Condition Characteristic signs and symptoms include confusion, disorientation, reduced ability to maintain or shift attention, fluctuation in level of consciousness, disorganized thinking, changes in activity level such as lethargy and/or agitation, memory impairment, perceptual disturbance/hallucinations, sleep-wake cycle disturbance, and emotional disturbance. The change from the patient's baseline profile is significant, and is most often severe. (see *DSM-IV* Criteria Appendix, p 311)	**Infancy and Early Childhood** Difficult to diagnose at this age. **Middle Childhood and Adolescence** The child and adolescent may demonstrate a reduced clarity of awareness of the environment, an inability to focus or sustain attention, or may be easily distracted by irrelevant stimuli or disoriented to time and place.

SPECIAL INFORMATION

There is little formal research on delirium in childhood. In infancy and early childhood, mild delirium is difficult to diagnose, especially in nonverbal patients; be alert to the possibility of accidental ingestions as the cause of delirium. In middle childhood, children are more verbal and delirium can more easily be diagnosed; be especially suspicious in medical settings and in children with previously diagnosed medical conditions. Delirious patients may be a risk to themselves or others and require close supervision. The individual's condition may fluctuate over the course of the day, seeming lucid and oriented at one point, but later demonstrating more obvious symptoms. Symptoms are commonly worse at night.

In young children, delirium may be misinterpreted as "naughty" behavior, or the associated agitation and emotional disturbance dismissed as an understandable reaction to illness and hospitalization. If familiar individuals cannot soothe the child, delirium may be the cause.

The clinician should not dismiss changes in mental status during a febrile illness as simply caused by fever, but instead should be alert to the real possibility that the illness producing the fever and confusion may be serious and potentially life threatening. This diagnosis can only be made after careful medical assessment and thoughtful workup.

DIFFERENTIAL DIAGNOSIS	SPECIAL INFORMATION

General Medical Conditions — Examples include:
Metabolic derangements:
  Hypoxia
  Hypoglycemia
  Acidosis
 	
Infections:
  Meningoencephalitis
  Human immunodeficiency virus
  Sepsis
 	
Endocrine disorders:
  Hypothyroidism
 	
Central nervous system disorders:
  Epilepsy
  Increased intracranial pressure
  Cerebrovascular disease
 	
Nutritional deficiency:
  B$_{12}$
 	
Systemic disease:
  Inflammatory diseases such as
    systemic lupus
	Delirium may be produced by any serious medical condition that is significantly advanced. The clinical picture of delirium should be considered to be the result of a nonpsychiatric medical disturbance until proven otherwise.
	
	The disorders discussed in the delirium section share a common symptom presentation of a disturbance in consciousness and cognition but are differentiated based on etiology:
	
	• Delirium due to a general medical condition (**293.0**)
	• Substance-induced delirium (**292.81**)
	• Delirium due to multiple etiologies
	• Delirium, not otherwise specified (**780.09**)
	
	Dementia is an acquired global impairment of intellect, memory, and personality that occurs without impairment of consciousness. It is uncommon, but not unheard of, in younger patients. An underlying physical etiology is assumed. Causes include inherited disorders associated with neurodegenerative processes such as Huntington's chorea, Niemann-Pick disease, and Wilson's disease, as well as toxins and infectious agents such as human immunodeficiency virus. Dementia may be distinguished from delirium in most cases by the relative preservation of consciousness and arousal, and a more chronic course.

Substances — Examples include: Alcohol Amphetamines and related substances Cocaine Cannabis Opioids Sedatives Hypnotics Anxiolytics Hallucinogens Phencyclidine Inhalants Drugs/toxins: Anticholinergics	Delirium may result from intoxication with a substance and may also result from withdrawal in some cases. For substances of abuse, code substance intoxication delirium or substance withdrawal delirium. Indicate the name of the substance (e.g., alcohol withdrawal delirium and code based on the specific substance involved). When a medication is causing the delirium, note it as _____ -induced delirium, giving the name of the medication, and code it as **292.81.**
Mental Disorders — Examples include: **295.xx** Schizophrenia **298.9** Psychotic disorder, not otherwise specified **296.x4** Mood disorder with psychotic features **290.xx, 294.x** Dementia **300.15** Dissociative disorder, not otherwise specified **V65.2** Malingering **300.16** Factitious disorder with predominantly psychological signs and symptoms **294.9** Cognitive disorder, not otherwise specified	The diagnosis of a primary psychiatric disorder as the cause for the clinical condition of a patient who appears delirious should be approached cautiously. Careful medical evaluation should take place prior to arriving at this conclusion.

COMMONLY COMORBID CONDITIONS	SPECIAL INFORMATION
Other Comorbid Mental Health Conditions — Examples include: **290.xx,** Dementia **294.x** **305.xx** Substance abuse **304.xx,** Substance dependence **303.xx** **319.** Unspecified mental retardation	Patients with disorders that affect the brain appear to be at especially high risk for delirium, particularly those with neurodegenerative disorders or dementia. Individuals with delirium may exhibit emotional disturbances such as anxiety, fear, depression, irritability, anger, euphoria, and apathy (see Sadness and Related Symptoms cluster, p 153 and Anxious Symptoms cluster, p 145).
Other General Medical Conditions — Examples include: Disturbance in sleep-wake cycle Disturbed psychomotor behavior Abnormal electroencephalogram findings	Virtually any preexisting medical condition may be associated with or predispose to delirium. Patients with structural brain disease may be at particularly high risk for delirium. Patients with preexisting medical conditions are also more likely to be taking medication that may also be a potential cause of delirium.

Appendix A

PRESENTING COMPLAINTS

Appendix B

Diagnostic Vignettes

Vignette 1

Clara, a 7-year-old girl in the 2nd grade at the Highstone Elementary School, is said to be shy and quiet and has few friends. Family acquaintances know that Clara is not so quiet at home. For years she has thrown temper tantrums at the slightest provocation.

It is hard to understand Clara's speech. She garbles her words and seems to get them in the wrong order. It's funny because she seems to be bright. She just doesn't talk the way her classmates do. This year, the children at school have started making jokes about Clara. They stand behind her, call her name, and then sputter at her. Their mimicry brings her to tears.

When Clara was small, she had seemed to understand everything that was said to her. She still does. But she took forever to start speaking. She was almost a year and a half before the family realized that she was calling their names. Her words were hard to understand even then. Adding common nouns and then verbs was also painfully slow. When she was 3, her mother would look into her face and know that Clara had something to say. The words just wouldn't come out.

She has had a tough time in nursery school and prekindergarten. She could match colors easily, but was the last child in the class to say "red" and "orange." She struggled with letter names. They just wouldn't come out. Sometimes she would pound her fist on the table.

Last year, Clara's parents were referred by their pediatrician to a speech and language pathologist and got a better idea about Clara's problems. She has an expressive language disorder and severely compromised articulation. She is now receiving therapy in school and her parents and teachers have received counseling about how the frustration Clara experiences can lead to the outbursts at home.

Impression:

> **315.31** Expressive Language Disorder
> **V71.02** Aggressive/Oppositional Problem

Discussion:

This child, with testing by the school speech clinician, has an expressive language problem. She also is demonstrating some oppositional and aggressive behaviors, suggesting some problems in her relationships with her parents and peers. These could be secondary to her language disorder and may improve as that disorder is addressed. At this point it is not severe enough to be considered a disorder.

Vignette 2

Terry is a 10-year-old boy who is struggling to keep up in the 4th grade at the Willothewisp School. He has trouble with reading and math. He cannot finish his classroom assignments in the time allotted for them. His teacher sends home his undone classroom papers in addition to his regular homework. Terry hates homework. He often cannot understand the written instructions and isn't sure where to begin. It is lucky that his younger sister Susan reads him the instructions out loud. He hopes the guys don't find out that an 8-year-old is helping him.

Terry loves sports and has lots of friends. He has no trouble following the coach's directions about complicated plays. But last week, he tried to read a book on soccer. Reading it took forever and it didn't make sense the way the coach does.

Terry can make change and do simple calculations in his head. But in class the written math problems are very hard for him. Even more challenging are the word problems. It takes him a long time to read the basic words, then to figure out the problem, and remember what it is he is supposed to do with the numbers. He really can't stand word problems.

Terry's dad is sympathetic but has just lost his job. He remembers well the challenges he and one of his brothers faced at the same age. He plugs for Terry and helps with homework when he gets home. He has written to the school district requesting that Terry's tests be untimed. He hopes that next year's teacher will have more training and experience teaching children with reading and math disabilities.

Impression:

> **V40.3** Learning Problem
> Suspected Reading Disorder (**315.00**) and possibly Mathematics Disorder (**315.1**)

Environmental Situations:

> **V62.0** Loss of Job

Discussion:

Terry has symptoms that suggest at least a reading disorder and possibly a mathematics disorder. Formal assessment of his general cognitive abilities and specific academic skills is needed to make a definitive diagnosis. In addition, he had the secondary stress of his father losing his job.

Vignette 3

Kevin is a good-looking 4-year-old. He is strong and runs gracefully. But something about Kevin is very odd. He just doesn't seem like other kids in the nursery class. He talks a lot, sometimes nonstop, but he doesn't join the circle time conversation. He is really "into" video movies like Aladdin and Beauty and the Beast. It is uncanny how he can recite whole passages from the movie. His voice is modulated like the characters, but not quite. He has an eery laugh.

And he doesn't look at you. It is almost as if you are not there, or worse, that you are a table or a chair. If you ask him, "Kevin, how are you?" the reply comes, "Kevin, how are you?" over and over as you try to make conversation with him. The echoed expressions ring in your ear and sound bizarre.

Is he a happy child? His parents say he dances and sings. He loves to play—but not with other children—with sand and water. He gets wound up in things. Very focused. He gets furious if he has to stop playing in the water to come to lunch.

He has strong dislikes. Loud noises bother him. He whines if his mother puts the wool sweater on him. He wriggles his neck to get away from the tag on his t-shirt. He complains about smells that are barely apparent to others.

He was an easy baby so all this difference and trouble are a surprise. Such an easy baby, but such a complex 4-year-old. The parents are very distressed about this problem and disagree about what to do. These disagreements intensify their ongoing marital problems.

Impression:

> Suspected **299.0** Autistic Disorder

Environmental Situations:

> **V61.20** Challenge to Primary Support Group
> **V61.1** Marital Discord

Discussion:

Kevin presents with a number of symptoms suggestive of autistic disorder and needs more extensive evaluation to make a definitive diagnosis. The symptoms are challenging his relationship with his parents and helping to create marital discord. This makes the need for evaluation and appropriate intervention all that more urgent.

Vignette 4

Michael, an 18-year-old male patient, has had spina bifida from birth. His lesion was at L1-L2, and he is wheelchair dependent. Through conditioning he had accomplished a bowel continence program in which he had deliberately developed a constipated stool pattern so that he could manually disimpact himself on a daily basis. He consults you because his bowels have become irregular and he has lately suffered some "accidents." However, his mood seems somewhat sad and he is not his usual animated self. The contrast is particularly striking in that you had seen him some 4 months before when he was anticipating beginning college and his first opportunity for independent living.

Further questioning reveals that the stresses of college have caused many of Michael's usual routines to be neglected. He had not been regularly disimpacting himself. It appeared that his "accident" was overflow incontinence. Unfortunately, it occurred when he was talking to a girl he particularly wanted to know better. Additionally, he found that independent living at college was more of a challenge than he had anticipated.

Impression:

> **316** Psychological Factors Affecting Medical Conditions
> **V40.3** Sadness Problem
> Adjustment Disorder (**309.xx**) needs to be ruled out (problem with adherence)
> Spina Bifida

Environmental Stressors:

> **V61.4** Chronic Health Condition
> **V62.4** Community or Social Challenges

Discussion:

Michael faces the challenge of a disability that can be made more challenging by the change in environment such as going off to college. He is manifesting a breakdown in his care and symptoms of a depressed mood. It is important to address his medical care program and determine if the depressed mood is more than at a problem level and may actually contribute to the non-compliance. Referral to a mental health clinician may be required to clarify this.

Vignette 5

Mrs. Smith, Allison's mother, consults you about the sudden onset of daytime urinary wetting. Allison is 4½ years old and had achieved both daytime and nighttime continence for 1 year. In the last 2 weeks, she has been wetting herself both at home and at nursery school; she has been enrolled in nursery school for about 1 year. You learn that the child's teacher retired over 1 month ago and has been replaced by another teacher. Allison's mother is also 4 months pregnant.

You conduct a physical exam that gives results completely within normal limits. A urinalysis is likewise normal and a urine culture is pending. An interview of the child indicates that she is excited about the upcoming birth of her sibling. Her mother reports that open visitation is encouraged at the school and due to cross-supervision; the likelihood of inappropriate sexual contact is remote.

Discussion with the nursery school teacher indicates that she feels that toileting issues at school are best handled on a "scheduled" basis so as not to interrupt "educational" opportunities at school.

Impression:

> **V40.3** Wetting Problem

Environmental Situations:

> **V61.20** Changes in Caregiving

Discussion:

Allison, who was previously dry, is now having accidents, causing her some difficulty in her preschool setting. She has to deal with a change in teachers as well as a rigid school bathroom schedule. Getting the teacher to allow for a more flexible system may resolve the problem. If it does not, the problem may need to be evaluated further.

Vignette 6

Jolene is a 15-year-old patient whom you have followed since age 6. She originally came to you at age 9 drinking approximately 2 gallons of water per day along with other fluids. Although you originally suspected psychogenic polydipsia, you were troubled by the patient's request that you help her so that she would no longer be forced to wake up at night to drink. Your evaluation shows that she had diabetes insipidus and a lesion of her pituitary. She was "cured" by resection of the pituitary and stalk, and began lifetime hormonal replacement therapy.

At age 11 she developed severe fatigue, for which no identifiable medical cause could be found. At age 12 she developed abdominal pain without an identifiable medical cause. At age 14 she developed knee and leg pain that proved to be reflex sympathetic dystrophy. She receives extensive physical therapy and treatment at a medical center pain program. She sees you because she has no energy, is "sick of seeing doctors," and appears depressed. During your evaluation, you repeat a physical and find her exam results to be at baseline; she is in the 75th percentile for height and 25th percentile for weight.

Impression:

> Rule out a mood disorder (**296.xx**)
> Rule out Bulimia Nervosa (**307.51**)
> General Medical Conditions:
> > Reflex Sympathetic Dystrophy
> > Panhypopituitarism
> > Diabetes Insipidus

Environmental Situations:

> **V61.4** Chronic Health Condition

Discussion:

Jolene has a long history of chronic health conditions and now presents with symptoms that suggest a mood disorder such as major depressive disorder. She requires referral to a mental health clinician for more extensive evaluation to determine the type and extent of the mood disorder or eating disorder, as well as a therapeutic plan.

Vignette 7

Corey's mother tells the pediatrician she is beginning to be concerned about the reports she receives from school that Corey, who is 6 years old, sometimes disrupts the classroom with talking out of turn and saying things that aren't related to what the class is doing. The parents have been concerned about Corey since about age 4 because he often seems "all wound up" and is difficult to settle for naps or at mealtimes. In addition, when he is asked to put away his toys or get ready for bed he sometimes becomes resistant and has temper tantrums. Sometimes babysitters have reported that they have a hard time getting him to get ready for bed, or to put away his things. Last year's kindergarten teacher reported that Corey was "high spirited" but felt he contributed to the class and was just "a little immature."

Corey is the first child of parents who both work "to make ends meet." A younger female sibling was born 2 years ago and the parents feel that Corey's problems really became apparent then. An added concern is the father's recent loss of job due to his company's downsizing. The mother continues to work full-time while the father is job hunting.

The teacher reports that Corey is learning to read and does average work in math. He particularly likes music and the teacher finds she can calm him down by playing music in the classroom.

Corey has a normal early medical history except for frequent ear infections between 18 months and 3 years of age. However, the last ear infection was a little more than 1 year ago and a hearing test then was normal.

Impression:

> **314.9** Hyperactive/Impulsive Behavior Problem
> **V61.8** Addition of a Sibling
> **V62.2** Loss of Job

Discussion:

From an early age Corey demonstrated hyperactive and impulsive symptoms. While they are causing some difficulties, at this point they do not appear severe enough to warrant a disorder diagnosis. Recent stressors such as the addition of a sibling and his father's job loss may be increasing the symptoms.

Vignette 8

Jimmy's mother tells the pediatrician that she's concerned about his hyperactive behavior. At 3½ years old, he has recently been enrolled in a nursery school for three half-days a week where the parents can stay if they wish. She notes that he runs around during the play sessions in circles and sometimes knocks over things. When the teacher tries to get them to snack time, he often wants "just one more" turn around the play area. At home sometimes he seems just to talk constantly and wants to ride his trike at "breakneck" speed. She has a hard time getting him to sleep at nap time because he's so wound up that he won't settle down. He sleeps well at night.

In the mornings, however, he'll sit at the kitchen table coloring and drawing for 20 minutes or more. When she sits him down to "read" a book, he loves turning the pages and pointing to the pictures that go with the story.

Jimmy is the first child of a professional couple. The mother was 35 and the father 36 when he was born. The mother now expresses concern about whether they should have another child.

On observation Jimmy is a very inquisitive child who asks constant questions while being examined. When the doctor tells him he can't play with the blood pressure cuff he responds by asking more questions but doesn't return to the pressure cuff. His physical and developmental assessment is normal to advanced.

The nursery school teacher is contacted and says, "Jimmy is a handful but he responds well to explanations and re-direction. He seems very bright." She does not feel that he is much more active than the other boys in his class.

Impression:

V65.4 Hyperactive/Impulsive Developmental Variation

Discussion:

Jimmy is an active preschooler with a high energy level. However, he functions reasonably well at home, school, and the physician's office. In addition, his teacher does not find him much different in his behavior than his peers. These are suggestive that his behaviors fit within the range of normal variations.

Vignette 9

"Jill seems less interested in her schoolwork and practicing the piano. Is this a phase? She's my first child to reach adolescence, and I don't know what to expect." On further history, Jill's mother noted that her daughter's appetite had decreased and she seemed to be staying up later at night, claiming to be unable to fall asleep. She seems more irritable and moody, choosing to spend more time in her room and less time with her 10-year-old sister. When asked by her mother, Jill says she just doesn't have much energy for either her schoolwork or for practicing like she used to. "What's most confusing, Doctor, is that she seems to go into these periods lasting a few days and then perks up." Overall, Jill, a 9th grader, is keeping up in school and in three other extracurricular activities. She had a best friend and mentioned had a "great time" in the local mall with a group of boys and girls from her class.

Jill is a well-appearing 14-year-old young woman, tanner stage 5, wearing rather somber but clean clothing and relating in a shy, gentle manner. Physical exam was unremarkable and a review of systems yielded no additional symptomatology. Jill answered that she had been feeling down at times, usually for periods lasting 2 or 3 days, and then she would seem to feel better and show more energy toward all of her activities. She was functioning well with her friends, enjoyed her piano lessons, and was a fullback on her freshman soccer team. She found the work at school somewhat more difficult, especially during her down moods, and her grades had dropped from the Bs to B- and one C. She noted that when she was down her appetite lessened, she had more trouble sleeping, and it was harder for her to concentrate. When asked if there was any pattern or trigger to her feeling down, she said that there were several, including when her mother got "down" on her for not helping around the house, when some of her friends leave her out of planned events, and whenever she got a poor grade in school. When asked about suicidal thoughts, Jill became more reluctant to talk but with encouragement noted that approximately a year ago she felt very down after her best friend moved away and did think what it would be like to be dead. However she quickly moved these thoughts out of her mind and since then has had no further suicidal ideation and remarked, "I would never do that."

Impression:

> At least a **V40.3** Sadness Problem but the possibility of a more extensive mood disorder needs to be further evaluated

Discussion:

Jill's withdrawal, at times to her room, tension with her mother's requests, and reactivity to situational events such as not being included by peers, is consistent with the variations associated with developing one's own identity and autonomy. However, the down mood, 2- to 3-day periods of withdrawal, irritability, during which there is a decreased appetite and difficulty sleeping are more consistent with a depressive disorder. At present it is not clear whether the symptoms meet criteria for a *DSM-IV* mood disorder, especially because they are of only several days' duration and in of themselves are not severe. Further evaluation is required to clarify the diagnosis.

Vignette 10

Cecilia is 22 months old. For most of her life she has had recurrent ear and upper respiratory infections—averaging one a month during her first winter and almost as many this winter. There is no evidence of an immune disorder or any deformity that might contribute to this tendency. Physically, her lungs have always been clear. There is no evidence of cardiovascular disease or dysfunction. Her growth has been consistently between the 25th and 50th percentiles. She is physically active, but makes few sounds, and speaks no words except "mama," "dada," and "ba" for bottle. She will only drink milk from the bottle and takes between 1½ and 2 quarts of milk per day. Treatment has been primarily with antibiotics. During both her first and second winter she received daily prophylaxis. Pneumatic otoscopy has been used to monitor the status of the middle ear: she has never had persistent fluid for more than 6 weeks. Her hearing was checked this year and was said to be normal by an audiologist.

Cecilia lives with both parents and two older siblings who are in school. There is a positive family history for allergy. Her father and her elder brother have had reading problems. Both parents are employed. Her mother has been very upset over the repeated infections. Cecilia cries throughout every office visit, no matter what the reason. She starts to scream in the parking lot, and continues uninterruptedly until the family leaves the building. She resists any attempt to be friendly, and struggles violently throughout the examination.

Impression:

> **316** Psychological Factors Affecting Medical Condition
> **V40.1** Speech/Language Problem
> Rule out Expressive Language Disorder (**315.31**)
> Rule out Mental Retardation (**317._, 318.x, 319**)
> Recurrent Otitis Media
> Possible Allergy to Milk or Other Allergic Rhinitis
> **V61.4** Chronic Health Condition

Discussion:

Cecilia's behaviors seem related to her medical experience with a health condition. While they are similar to negative emotional behaviors, the fact that they only occur secondary to medical encounters suggest the former diagnosis. Given her history of possible hearing loss secondary to chronic otitis and her delay in development, it is very important to assess and monitor her cognitive and language status.

Appendix C

SECTIONS OF THE RELEVANT CRITERIA OF THE DIAGNOSTIC AND STATISTICAL MANUAL OF MENTAL DISORDERS (DSM-IV)

The purpose of this appendix is to provide details on the diagnostic categories for the *DSM-IV* disorders pertinent to children. The disorders are listed in alphabetical order.

◆ Diagnostic criteria for Acute Stress Disorder 308.3

A. The person has been exposed to a traumatic event in which both of the following were present:
   (1) the person experienced, witnessed, or was confronted with an event or events that involved actual or threatened death or serious injury, or a threat to the physical integrity of self or others
   (2) the person's response involved intense fear, helplessness, or horror

B. Either while experiencing or after experiencing the distressing event, the individual has three (or more) of the following dissociative symptoms:
   (1) a subjective sense of numbing, detachment, or absence of emotional responsiveness
   (2) a reduction in awareness of his or her surroundings (e.g., "being in a daze")
   (3) derealization
   (4) depersonalization
   (5) dissociative amnesia (i.e., inability to recall an important aspect of the trauma)

C. The traumatic event is persistently reexperienced in at least one of the following ways: recurrent images, thoughts, dreams, illusions, flashback episodes, or a sense of reliving the experience, or distress on exposure to reminders of the traumatic event.

D. Marked avoidance of stimuli that arouse recollections of the trauma (e.g., thoughts, feelings, conversations, activities, places, people).

E. Marked symptoms of anxiety or increased arousal (e.g., difficulty sleeping, irritability, poor concentration, hypervigilance, exaggerated startle response, motor restlessness).

F. The disturbance causes clinically significant distress or impairment in social, occupational, or other important areas of functioning, or impairs the individual's ability to pursue some necessary task, such as obtaining necessary assistance or mobilizing personal resources by telling family members about the traumatic experience.

G. The disturbance lasts for a minimum of 2 days and a maximum of 4 weeks and occurs within 4 weeks of the traumatic event.

H. The disturbance is not due to the direct physiological effects of a substance (e.g., a drug, a medication) or a general medical condition.

◆ Diagnostic criteria for Adjustment Disorders 309.__

A. The development of emotional or behavioral symptoms in response to an identifiable stressor(s) occurring within 3 months of the onset of the stressor(s).

B. These symptoms or behaviors are clinically significant as evidenced by either of the following:
   (1) marked distress that is in excess of what would be expected from exposure to the stressor
   (2) significant impairment in social or occupational (academic) functioning

C. The stress-related disturbance does not meet the criteria for another specific disorder and is not merely an exacerbation of a preexisting disorder.

D. The symptoms do not represent bereavement.

E. Once the stressor (or its consequences) has terminated, the symptoms do not persist for more than an additional 6 months.

Specify if:

Acute: if the disturbance lasts less than 6 months
Chronic: if the disturbance lasts for 6 months or longer adjustment disorders are coded based on the subtype, which is selected according to the predominant symptoms.

309.0   With Depressed Mood
309.24 With Anxiety
309.28 With Mixed Anxiety and Depressed Mood
309.3   With Disturbance of Conduct
309.4   With Mixed Disturbance of Emotions and Conduct
309.9   Unspecified

Subtypes and Specifiers

Adjustment disorders are coded according to the subtype that best characterizes the predominant symptoms:

309.0 With Depressed Mood. This subtype should be used when the predominant manifestations are symptoms such as depressed mood, tearfulness, or feelings of hopelessness.

309.24 With Anxiety. This subtype should be used when the predominant manifestations are symptoms such as nervousness, worry, jitteriness or, in children, fears of separation from major attachment figures.

309.28 With Mixed Anxiety and Depressed Mood. This subtype should be used when the predominant manifestation is a combination of depression and anxiety.

309.3 With Disturbance of Conduct. This subtype should be used when the predominant manifestation is a disturbance in conduct in which there is violation of the rights of others or of major age-appropriate societal norms and rules (e.g., truancy, vandalism, reckless driving, fighting, defaulting on legal responsibilities).

309.4 With Mixed Disturbance of Emotions and Conduct. This subtype should be used when the predominant manifestations are both emotional symptoms (e.g., depression, anxiety) and a disturbance of conduct (see above subtype).

309.9   Unspecified. This subtype should be used for maladaptive reactions (e.g., physical complaints, social withdrawal, or work or academic inhibition) to psychosocial stressors that are not classifiable as one of the specific subtypes of adjustment disorder.

The duration of the symptoms of an adjustment disorder can be indicated by choosing one of the following specifiers:

Acute. This specifier can be used to indicate persistence of symptoms for less than 6 months.

Chronic. This specifier can be used to indicate persistence of symptoms for 6 months or longer. By definition, symptoms cannot persist for more than 6 months after the termination of the stressor or its consequences. The chronic specifier therefore applies when the duration of the disturbance is longer than 6 months in response to a chronic stressor or to a stressor that has enduring consequences.

◆ Diagnostic criteria for Anorexia Nervosa 307.1 (see Dieting/Body Image Problems Cluster, p 227)

◆ Diagnostic criteria for Antisocial Personality Disorder 301.7

A. There is a pervasive pattern of disregard for and violation of the rights of others occurring since age 15 years, as indicated by three (or more) of the following:

    (1)   failure to conform to social norms with respect to lawful behaviors as indicated by repeatedly performing acts that are grounds for arrest

    (2)   deceitfulness, as indicated by repeated lying, use of aliases, or conning others for personal profit or pleasure

    (3)   impulsivity or failure to plan ahead

    (4)   irritability and aggressiveness, as indicated by repeated physical fights or assaults

    (5)   reckless disregard for safety of self or others

    (6)   consistent irresponsibility, as indicated by repeated failure to sustain consistent work behavior or honor financial obligations

    (7)   lack of remorse, as indicated by being indifferent or rationalizing having hurt, mistreated, or stolen from another

B. The individual is at least age 18 years.

C. There is evidence of conduct disorder with onset before age 15 years.

D. The occurrence of antisocial behavior is not exclusively during the course of schizophrenia or a manic episode.

◆ Diagnostic criteria for Anxiety Disorder Due To...(*Indicate a General Medical Condition*) 293.84

A. Prominent anxiety, panic attacks, or obsessions or compulsions predominate in the clinical picture.

B. There is evidence from the history, physical examination, or laboratory findings that the disturbance is the direct physiological consequence of a general medical condition.

C. The disturbance is not better accounted for by another mental disorder (e.g., adjustment disorder with anxiety in which the stressor is a serious general medical condition).

D. The disturbance does not occur exclusively during the course of a delirium.

E. The disturbance causes clinically significant distress or impairment in social, occupational, or other important areas of functioning.

Specify if:

With Generalized Anxiety: if excessive anxiety or worry about a number of events or activities predominates in the clinical presentation

With Panic Attacks: if panic attacks predominate in the clinical presentation

With Obsessive-Compulsive Symptoms: if obsessions or compulsions predominate in the clinical presentation

Coding note: Include the name of the general medication condition, e.g., **316** anxiety disorder due to pheochromocytoma.

◆ Diagnostic criteria for Anxiety Disorder, Not Otherwise Specified 300.00

This category includes disorders with prominent anxiety or phobic avoidance that do not meet criteria for any specific anxiety disorder, adjustment disorder with anxiety, or adjustment disorder with mixed anxiety and depressed mood. Examples include:

(1) Mixed anxiety-depressive disorder: clinically significant symptoms of anxiety and depression, but the criteria are not met for either a specific mood disorder or a specific anxiety disorder

(2) Clinically significant social phobic symptoms that are related to the social impact of having a general medical condition or mental disorder (e.g., Parkinson's disease, dermatological conditions, stuttering, anorexia nervosa, body dysmorphic disorder)

(3) Situations in which the clinician has concluded that an anxiety disorder is present but is unable to determine whether it is primary, due to a general medical condition, or substance induced

◆ Diagnostic criteria for Asperger's Disorder 299.80

A. Qualitative impairment in social interaction, as manifested by at least two of the following:
   (1) marked impairment in the use of multiple nonverbal behaviors such as eye-to-eye gaze, facial expression, body postures, and gestures to regular social interaction
   (2) failure to develop peer relationships appropriate to developmental level
   (3) a lack of spontaneous seeking to share enjoyment, interests, or achievements with other people (e.g., by a lack of showing, bringing, or pointing out objects of interest to other people)
   (4) lack of social or emotional reciprocity

B. Restricted repetitive and stereotyped patterns of behavior, interests, and activities, as manifested by at least one of the following:
   (1) encompassing preoccupation with one or more stereotyped and restricted patterns of interest that is abnormal either in intensity or focus
   (2) apparently inflexible adherence to specific, nonfunctional routines or rituals
   (3) stereotyped and repetitive motor mannerisms (e.g., hand or finger flapping or twisting, or complex whole-body movements)
   (4) persistent preoccupation with parts of objects

C. The disturbance causes clinically significant impairment in social, occupational, or other important areas of functioning.

D. There is no clinically significant general delay in language (e.g., single words used by 2 years, communicative phrases used by age 3 years).

E. There is no clinically significant delay in cognitive development or in the development of age-appropriate self-help skills, adaptive behavior (other than in social interaction), and curiosity about the environment in childhood.

F. Criteria are not met for another specific pervasive developmental disorder or schizophrenia.

◆ Diagnostic criteria for Attention-Deficit/Hyperactivity Disorder Combined Type 314.01 (see Hyperactive/Impulsive Behaviors cluster, p 93).

◆ Diagnostic criteria for Attention-Deficit/Hyperactivity Disorder Predominantly Hyperactive-Impulsive Type 314.01 (see Hyperactive/Impulsive Behavior cluster, p 93).

◆ **Diagnostic criteria for Attention-Deficit/Hyperactivity Disorder Predominantly Inattentive Type 314.00 (see Inattentive Behaviors cluster, p 103).**

◆ **Diagnostic criteria for Attention-Deficit/Hyperactivity Disorder, Not Otherwise Specified 314.9**

This category is for disorders with prominent symptoms of inattention or hyperactivity-impulsivity that do not meet criteria for attention-deficit/hyperactivity disorder.

◆ **Diagnostic criteria for Autistic Disorder 299.00**

A. A total of six (or more) items from (1), (2), and (3), with at least two from (1), and one each from (2) and (3):

(1) qualitative impairment in social interaction, as manifested by at least two of the following:

(a) marked impairment in the use of multiple nonverbal behaviors such as eye-to-eye gaze, facial expression, body postures, and gestures to regular social interaction

(b) failure to develop peer relationship appropriate to developmental level

(c) a lack of spontaneous seeking to share enjoyment, interests, or achievements with other people (e.g., by a lack of showing, bringing, or pointing out objects of interest)

(d) lack of social or emotional reciprocity

(2) qualitative impairments in communication as manifested by at least one of the following:

(a) delay in, or total lack of, the development of spoken language (not accompanied by an attempt to compensate through alternative modes of communication such as gesture or mime)

(b) in individuals with adequate speech, marked impairment in the ability to initiate or sustain a conversation with others

(c) stereotyped and repetitive use of language or idiosyncratic language

(d) lack of varied, spontaneous make-believe play or social imitative play appropriate to developmental level

(3) restricted repetitive and stereotyped patterns of behavior, interests, and activities, as manifested by at least one of the following:

(a) encompassing preoccupation with one or more stereotyped and restricted patterns of interest that is abnormal either in intensity or focus

(b) apparently inflexible adherence to specific, nonfunctional routines or rituals

(c) stereotyped and repetitive motor mannerisms (e.g., hand or finger flapping or twisting, or complex whole-body movements)

(d) persistent preoccupation with parts of objects

B. Delays or abnormal functioning in at least one of the following areas, with onset prior to age 3 years: (1) social interaction, (2) language as used in social communication, or (3) symbolic or imaginative play.

C. The disturbance is not better accounted for by Rett's disorder or childhood disintegrative disorder.

◆ Diagnostic criteria for Avoidant Personality Disorder 301.82

A pervasive pattern of social inhibition, feelings of inadequacy, and hypersensitivity to negative evaluation, beginning by early adulthood, and present in a variety of contexts, as indicated by four (or more) of the following:

(1) avoids occupational activities that involve significant interpersonal contact because of fears of criticism, disapproval, or rejection

(2) is unwilling to get involved with people unless certain of being liked

(3) shows restraint within intimate relationships because of the fear of being shamed or ridiculed

(4) is preoccupied with being criticized or rejected in social situations

(5) is inhibited in new interpersonal situations because of feelings of inadequacy

(6) views self as socially inept, personally unappealing, or inferior to others

(7) is unusually reluctant to take personal risks or to engage in any new activities because they may prove embarrassing

◆ Diagnostic criteria for Bipolar I Disorder, Most Recent Episode Depressed 296.5x

A. Currently (or most recently) in a major depressive episode.

B. There has previously been at least one manic episode or mixed episode.

C. The mood episodes in criteria A and B are not better accounted for by schizoaffective disorder and are not superimposed on schizophrenia, schizophreniform disorder, delusional disorder, or psychotic disorder not otherwise specified.

Specify (for current or most recent episode):

Severity/Psychotic/Remission Specifiers

296.56 In full remission

296.55 In partial remission

296.51 Mild

296.52 Moderate

296.53 Severe without psychotic features

296.54 Severe with psychotic features

296.50 Unspecified

◆ Diagnostic criteria for Bipolar I Disorder, Most Recent Episode Hypomanic 296.40

A. Currently (or most recently) in a hypomanic episode.

B. There has previously been at least one manic episode or mixed episode.

C. The mood symptoms cause clinically significant distress or impairment in social, occupational, or other important areas of functioning.

D. The mood episodes in criteria A and B are not better accounted for by schizoaffective disorder and are not superimposed on schizophrenia, schizophreniform disorder, delusional disorder, or psychotic disorder not otherwise specified.

Specify (for current or most recent episode):

296.46 In full remission
296.45 In partial remission
296.41 Mild

◆ Diagnostic criteria for Bipolar I Disorder, Most Recent Episode Manic 296.4x

A. Currently (or most recently) in a manic episode.

B. There has previously been at least one major depressive episode, manic episode, or mixed episode.

C. The mood episodes in criteria A and B are not better accounted for by schizoaffective disorder and are not superimposed on schizophrenia, schizophreniform disorder, delusional disorder, or psychotic disorder not otherwise specified.

Specify (for current or most recent episode):

Severity/Psychotic/Remission Specifiers
296.46 In full remission
296.45 In partial remission
296.41 Mild
296.42 Moderate
296.43 Severe Without Psychotic Features
296.44 Severe With Psychotic Features
296.40 Unspecified

◆ Diagnostic criteria for Bipolar I Disorder, Most Recent Episode Mixed 296.6x

A. Currently (or most recently) in a mixed episode.

B. There has previously been at least one major depressive episode, manic episode, or mixed episode.

C. The mood episodes in criteria A and B are not better accounted for by schizoaffective disorder and are not superimposed on schizophrenia, schizophreniform disorder, delusional disorder, or psychotic disorder not otherwise specified.

Specify (for current or most recent episode):

296.66 In full remission
296.65 In partial remission
296.61 Mild
296.62 Moderate
296.63 Severe Without Psychotic Features
296.64 Severe With Psychotic Features
296.60 Unspecified

◆ Diagnostic criteria for Bipolar I Disorder, Single Manic Episode 296.0x

A. Presence of only one manic episode and no past major depressive episodes. **Note:** Recurrence is defined as either a change in polarity from depression or an interval of at least 2 months without manic symptoms.

B. The manic episode is not better accounted for by schizoaffective disorder and is not superimposed on schizophrenia, schizophreniform disorder, delusional disorder, or psychotic disorder, not otherwise specified.

Specify if:

Mixed: if symptoms meet criteria for a mixed episode.

Specify (for current or most recent episode):

Severity/Psychotic/Remission Specifiers
    296.06 In full remission
    296.05 In partial remission
    296.01 Mild
    296.02 Moderate
    296.03 Severe Without Psychotic Features
    296.04 Severe With Psychotic Features
    296.00 Unspecified

◆ Diagnostic criteria for Body Dysmorphic Disorder 300.7

A. Preoccupation with an imagined defect in appearance. If a slight physical anomaly is present, the person's concern is markedly excessive.

B. The preoccupation causes clinically significant distress or impairment in social, occupational, or other important areas of functioning.

C. The preoccupation is not better accounted for by another mental disorder (e.g., dissatisfaction with body shape and size in anorexia nervosa).

◆ Diagnostic criteria for Borderline Personality Disorder 301.83

A pervasive pattern of instability of interpersonal relationships, self-image, and affects, and marked impulsivity beginning by early adulthood and present in a variety of contexts, as indicated by five (or more) of the following:

(1) frantic efforts to avoid real or imagined abandonment. **Note:** Do not include suicidal or self-mutilating behavior covered in criterion 5.

(2) a pattern of unstable and intense interpersonal relationships characterized by alternating between extremes of idealization and devaluation

(3) identity disturbance: markedly and persistently unstable self-image or sense of self

(4) impulsivity in at least two areas that are potentially self-damaging (e.g., spending, sex, substance abuse, reckless, driving, binge eating). **Note:** Do not include suicidal or self-mutilating behavior covered in criterion 5.

(5) recurrent suicidal behavior, gestures, or threats, or self-mutilating behavior

(6) affective instability due to a marked reactivity of mood (e.g., intense episodic dysphoria, irritability, or anxiety usually lasting a few hours and only rarely more than a few days)

(7) chronic feelings of emptiness

(8) inappropriate, intense anger or difficulty controlling anger (e.g., frequent displays of temper, constant anger, recurrent physical fights)

(9) transient, stress-related paranoid ideation or severe dissociative symptoms

◆ Diagnostic criteria for Breathing-Related Sleep Disorder 780.59

A. Sleep disruption, leading to excessive sleepiness or insomnia, that is judged to be due to a sleep-related breathing condition (e.g., obstructive or central sleep apnea syndrome or central alveolar hypoventilation syndrome).

B. The disturbance is not better accounted for by another mental disorder and is not due to the direct physiological effects of a substance (e.g., a drug of abuse, a medication) or another general medical condition (other than a breathing-related disorder).

◆ Diagnostic criteria for Bulimia Nervosa 307.51 (see Purging/ Binge-Eating cluster, p 221)

◆ Diagnostic criteria for Childhood Disintegrative Disorder 299.10

A. Apparently normal development for at least the first 2 years after birth as manifested by the presence of age-appropriate verbal and nonverbal communication, social relationships, play, and adaptive behavior.

B. Clinically significant loss of previously acquired skills (before age 10 years) in at least two of the following areas:

   (1) expressive or receptive language

   (2) social skills or adaptive behavior

   (3) bowel or bladder control

   (4) play

   (5) motor skills

C. Abnormalities of functioning in at least two of the following areas:

   (1) qualitative impairment in social interaction (e.g., impairment in nonverbal behaviors, failure to develop peer relationships, lack of social or emotional reciprocity)

   (2) qualitative impairments in communication (e.g., delay or lack of spoken language, inability to initiate or sustain a conversation, stereotyped and repetitive use of language, lack of varied make-believe play)

   (3) restricted, repetitive, and stereotyped patterns of behavior, interests, and activities, including motor stereotypies and mannerisms

D. The disturbance is not better accounted for by another specific pervasive developmental disorder or by schizophrenia.

◆ Diagnostic criteria for Chronic Motor or Vocal Tic Disorder 307.22 (see Repetitive Behavioral Patterns cluster, p 269)

◆ Diagnostic criteria for Circadian Rhythm Sleep Disorder 307.45

A. A persistent or recurrent pattern of sleep disruption leading to excessive sleepiness or insomnia that is due to a mismatch between the sleep-wake schedule required by a person's environment and his or her circadian sleep-wake pattern.

B. The sleep disturbance causes clinically significant distress or impairment in social, occupational, or other important areas of functioning.

C. The disturbance does not occur exclusively during the course of another sleep disorder or other mental disorder.

D. The disturbance is not due to the direct physiological effects of a substance (e.g., a drug of abuse, a medication) or a general medical condition.

Specify type:

Delayed Sleep Phase Type: a persistent pattern of late sleep onset and late awakening times, with an inability to fall asleep and awaken at a desired earlier time

Jet Lag Type: sleepiness and alertness that occur at an inappropriate time of day relative to local time, occurring after repeated travel across more than one time zone

Shift Work Type: insomnia during the major sleep period or excessive sleepiness during the major awake period associated with night shift work or frequently changing shift work

Unspecified Type

◆ Diagnostic criteria for Communication Disorder, Not Otherwise Specified 307.9

This category is for disorders in communication that do not meet criteria for any specific communication disorder, for example, a voice disorder (i.e., an abnormality of vocal pitch, loudness, quality, tone, or resonance).

◆ Diagnostic criteria for Conduct Disorder 312.81 and 312.82

A. A repetitive and persistent pattern in which the basic rights of others or major age-appropriate societal norms or rules are violated, as manifested by the presence of three (or more) of the following criteria in the past 12 months, with at least one criterion present in the past 6 months.

Aggression to people and animals
(1) often bullies, threatens, or intimidates others
(2) often initiates physical fights
(3) has used a weapon that can cause serious physical harm to others (e.g., a bat, brick, broken bottle, knife, gun)
(4) has been physically cruel to people
(5) has been physically cruel to animals
(6) has stolen while confronting a victim (e.g., mugging, purse snatching, extortion, armed robbery)
(7) has forced someone into sexual activity

Destruction of property
(8) has deliberately engaged in fire setting with the intention of causing serious damage
(9) has deliberately destroyed others' property (other than by fire setting)

Deceitfulness or theft
(10) has broken into someone else's house, building, or car
(11) often lies to obtain goods or favors or to avoid obligations (i.e., "cons" others)

(12) has stolen items of nontrivial value without confronting a victim (e.g., shoplifting, but without breaking and entering; forgery)

Serious violations of rules

(13) often stays out at night despite parental prohibitions, beginning before age 13 years

(14) has run away from home overnight at least twice while living in parental or parental surrogate home (or once without returning for a lengthy period)

(15) is often truant from school, beginning before age 13 years

B. The disturbance in behavior causes clinically significant impairment in social, academic, or occupational functioning.

C. If the individual is age 18 years or older, criteria are not met for antisocial personality disorder.

Specify type based on age at onset:

Childhood-Onset Type: onset of at least one criterion characteristic of conduct disorder prior to age 10 years

Adolescent-Onset Type: absence of any criteria characteristic of conduct disorder prior to age 10 years

Specify severity:

Mild: few if any conduct problems in excess of those required to make the diagnosis and conduct problems cause only minor harm to others

Moderate: number of conduct problems and effect on others intermediate between "mild" and "severe"

Severe: many conduct problems in excess of those required to make the diagnosis or conduct problems cause considerable harm to others

◆ Diagnostic criteria for Conversion Disorder 300.11

A. One or more symptoms or deficits affecting voluntary motor or sensory function that suggest a neurological or other general medical condition.

B. Psychological factors are judged to be associated with the symptom or deficit because the initiation or exacerbation of the symptom or deficit is preceded by conflicts or other stressors.

C. The symptom or deficit is not intentionally produced or feigned (as in factitious disorder or malingering).

D. The symptom or deficit cannot, after appropriate investigation, be fully explained by a general medical condition, or by the direct effects of a substance, or as a culturally sanctioned behavior or experience.

E. The symptom or deficit causes clinically significant distress or impairment in social, occupational, or other important areas of functioning or warrants medical evaluation.

F. The symptom or deficit is not limited to pain or sexual dysfunction, does not occur exclusively during the course of somatization disorder, and is not better accounted for by another mental disorder.

Specify **type of symptom or deficit:**

With Motor Symptom or Deficit
With Sensory Symptom or Deficit
With Seizures or Convulsions
With Mixed Presentation

◆ Diagnostic criteria for Cyclothymic Disorder 301.13

A. For at least 2 years, the presence of numerous periods with hypomanic symptoms and numerous periods with depressive symptoms that do not meet criteria for a major depressive episode. **Note:** In children and adolescents, the duration must be at least 1 year.

B. During the above 2-year period (1 year in children and adolescents), the person has not been without the symptoms in criterion A for more than 2 months at a time.

C. No major depressive episode, manic episode, or mixed episode has been present during the first 2 years of the disturbance. **Note:** After the initial 2 years (1 year in children and adolescents) of cyclothymic disorder, there may be superimposed manic or mixed episodes (in which case both bipolar II disorder and cyclothymic disorder may be diagnosed).

D. The symptoms in criterion A are not better accounted for by schizoaffective disorder and are not superimposed on schizophrenia, schizophreniform disorder, delusional disorder, or psychotic disorder, not otherwise specified.

E. The symptoms are not due to the direct physiological effects of a substance (e.g., a drug of abuse, a medication) or a general medical condition (e.g., hyperthyroidism).

F. The symptoms cause clinically significant distress or impairment in social, occupational, or other important areas of functioning.

◆ Diagnostic criteria for Delirium Due To...(*Indicate the General Medical Condition*) 293.0

A. Disturbance of consciousness (i.e., reduced clarity of awareness of the environment) with reduced ability to focus, sustain, or shift attention

B. A change in cognition (such as memory deficit, disorientation, language disturbance) or the development of a perceptual disturbance that is not better accounted for by a preexisting, established, or evolving dementia.

C. The disturbance develops over a short period of time (usually hours to days) and tends to fluctuate during the course of the day.

D. There is evidence from the history, physical examination, or laboratory findings that the disturbance is caused by the direct physiological consequences of a general medical condition.

Coding note: If delirium is superimposed on a preexisting dementia of the Alzheimer's type or vascular dementia, indicate the delirium by coding the appropriate subtype of the dementia, e.g., **290.3** Dementia of the Alzheimer's Type, With Late Onset, With Delirium. **Coding note:** Include the name of the general medical condition, e.g., **293.0** Delirium Due To Hepatic Encephalopathy.

◆ Diagnostic criteria for Developmental Coordination Disorder 315.4 (see Motor Development cluster, p 77).

◆ Diagnostic criteria for Disorder of Written Expression 315.2 (see Academic Skills cluster, p 69).

◆ Diagnostic criteria for Disruptive Behavior Disorder, Not Otherwise Specified 312.9

This category is for disorders characterized by conduct or oppositional defiant behaviors that do not meet the criteria for conduct disorder or oppositional defiant disorder. For example, include clinical presentations that do not meet full criteria either for oppositional defiant disorder or conduct disorder, but in which there is clinically significant impairment.

◆ Diagnostic criteria for Dyssomnia, Not Otherwise Specified 307.47

The Dyssomnia, Not Otherwise Specified category is for insomnias, hypersomnias, or circadian rhythm disturbances that do not meet criteria for any specific dyssomnia. Examples include:

1. Complaints of clinically significant insomnia or hypersomnia that are attributable to environmental factors (e.g., noise, light, frequent interruptions).

2. Excessive sleepiness that is attributable to ongoing sleep deprivation.

3. Idiopathic "Restless Legs Syndrome": uncomfortable sensations (e.g., discomfort, crawling sensations, or restlessness) that lead to an intense urge to move the legs. Typically, the sensations begin in the evening before sleep onset and are temporarily relieved by moving the legs or walking, only to begin again when the legs are immobile. The sensations can delay sleep onset or awaken the individual from sleep.

4. Idiopathic periodic limb movements ("nocturnal myoclonus"): repeated low-amplitude brief limb jerks, particularly in the lower extremities. These movements begin near sleep onset and decrease during stage 3 or 4 non-rapid eye movement (NREM) and rapid eye movement (REM) sleep. Movements usually occur rhythmically every 20–60 seconds, leading to repeated, brief arousals. Individuals are typically unaware of the actual movements, but may complain of insomnia, frequent awakenings, or daytime sleepiness if the number of movements is very large.

5. Situations in which the clinician has concluded that a dyssomnia is present but is unable to determine whether it is primary, due to a general medical condition, or substance induced.

◆ Diagnostic criteria for Dysthymic Disorder 300.4

A. Depressed mood for most of the day, for more days than not, as indicated either by subjective account or observation by others, for at least 2 years. **Note:** In children and adolescents, mood can be irritable and duration must be at least 1 year.

B. Presence, while depressed, of two (or more) of the following:
   (1) poor appetite or overeating
   (2) insomnia or hypersomnia
   (3) low energy or fatigue
   (4) low self-esteem
   (5) poor concentration or difficulty making decisions
   (6) feelings of hopelessness

C. During the 2-year period (2 year for children or adolescents) of the disturbance, the person has never been without the symptoms in criteria A and B for more than 2 months at a time.

D. No major depressive episode has been present during the first 2 years of the disturbance (1 year for children and adolescents); i.e., the disturbance is not better accounted for by chronic major depressive disorder, or major depressive disorder, or major depressive disorder, in partial remission. **Note:** There may have been a previous major depressive episode provided there was a full remission (no significant signs or symptoms for 2 months) before development of the dysthymic disorder. In addition, after the initial 2 years (1 year in children or adolescents) of dysthymic disorder, there may be superimposed episodes of major depressive disorder, in which case both diagnoses may be given when the criteria are met for a major depressive episode.

E. There has never been a manic episode, a mixed episode, or a hypomanic episode, and criteria have never been met for cyclothymic disorder.

F. The disturbance does not occur exclusively during the course of a chronic psychotic disorder, such as schizophrenia or delusional disorder.

G. The symptoms are not due to the direct physiological effects of a substance (e.g., a drug of abuse, a medication), or a general medical condition (e.g., hypothyroidism).

H. The symptoms cause clinically significant distress or impairment in social, occupational, or other important areas of functioning.

Specify if:

Early Onset: if onset is before age 21 years

Late Onset: if onset is age 21 or older

Specify (for most recent 2 years of dysthymic disorder):
With Atypical Features

◆ Diagnostic criteria for Eating Disorder, Not Otherwise Specified 307.50

The Eating Disorder, Not Otherwise Specified category is for disorders of eating that do not meet the criteria for any specific eating disorder. Examples include:

1. For females, all of the criteria for anorexia nervosa are met except that the individual has regular menses

2. All of the criteria for anorexia nervosa are met except that, despite significant weight loss, the individual's current weight is in the normal range

3. All of the criteria for bulimia nervosa are met except that the binge eating and inappropriate compensatory mechanisms occur at a frequency of less than twice a week or for a duration of less than 3 months

4. The regular use of inappropriate compensatory behavior by an individual of normal body weight after eating small amounts of food (e.g., self-induced vomiting after the consumption of two cookies)

5. Repeatedly chewing and spitting out, but not swallowing, large amounts of food

6. Binge-eating disorder: recurrent episodes of binge eating in the absence of the regular use of inappropriate compensatory behaviors characteristic of bulimia nervosa

◆ Diagnostic criteria for Encopresis With Constipation Overflow Incontinence 787.6 (see Soiling Problem cluster, p 209).

◆ Diagnostic criteria for Encopresis Without Constipation and Overflow Incontinence 307.7 (see Soiling Problem cluster, p 209).

◆ Diagnostic criteria for Enuresis 307.6 (see Day/Nighttime Wetting Problem cluster, p 215).

◆ **Diagnostic criteria for Expressive Language Disorder 315.31 (see Speech and Language cluster, p 83).**

◆ **Diagnostic criteria for Factitious disorder 300.xx**

A. Intentional production or feigning of physical or psychological signs or symptoms.
B. The motivation for the behavior is to assume the sick role.
C. External incentives for the behavior (such as economic gain, avoiding legal responsibility, or improving physical well-being, as in malingering) are absent.

Code **based on type:**

300.16 With Predominantly Psychological Signs and Symptoms: if psychological signs and symptoms predominate in the clinical presentation

300.19 With Predominantly Physical Signs and Symptoms: if physical signs and symptoms predominate in the clinical presentation

300.19 With Combined Psychological and Physical Signs and Symptoms: if both psychological and physical signs and symptoms are present but neither predominates in the clinical presentation

◆ **Diagnostic criteria for Factitious Disorder, Not Otherwise Specified 300.19**

This category includes disorders with factitious symptoms that do not meet the criteria for factitious disorder. An example is factitious disorder by proxy: the intentional production or feigning of physical or psychological signs or symptoms in another person who is under the individual's care for the purpose of indirectly assuming the sick role (see p.725 for suggested research criteria).

◆ **Diagnostic criteria for Feeding Disorder of Infancy or Early Childhood 307.59 (see Irregular Feeding Behaviors Cluster, p 235).**

◆ **Diagnostic criteria for Gender Identity Disorder 302.85**

A. A strong and persistent cross-gender identification (not merely a desire for any perceived cultural advantages of being the other sex). In children, the disturbance is manifested by four (or more) of the following:
   (1) repeatedly stated desire to be, or insistence that he or she is, the other sex
   (2) in boys, preference for cross-dressing or simulating female attire; in girls, insistence on wearing only stereotypical masculine clothing
   (3) strong and persistent fantasies of being the other sex
   (4) intense desire to participate in the stereotypical games and pastimes of the other sex

(5) strong preference for playmates of the other sex. In adolescence and adults, the disturbance is manifested by symptoms such as a stated desire to be the other sex, frequent passing as the other sex, desire to live or be treated as the other sex, or the conviction that he or she has the typical feelings and reactions of the other sex.

B. Persistent discomfort with his or her sex or sense of inappropriateness in the gender role of that sex.

In children, the disturbance is manifested by any of the following: in boys, assertion that his penis or testes are disgusting or will disappear or assertion that it would be better not to have a penis, or aversion toward rough-and-tumble play and rejection of male stereotypical toys, games, and activities; in girls, rejection of urinating in a sitting position, assertion that she has or will grow a penis, or assertion that she does not want to grow breasts or menstruate, or marked aversion toward normative feminine clothing.

In adolescents and adults, the disturbance is manifested by symptoms such as preoccupation with getting rid of primary and secondary sex characteristics (e.g., request for hormones, surgery, or other procedures to physically alter sexual characteristics to simulate the other sex) or belief that he or she was born the wrong sex.

C. The disturbance is not concurrent with a physical intersex condition.

D. The disturbance causes clinically significant distress or impairment in social, occupational, or other important areas of functioning.

Code **based on current age:**

302.6   Gender Identity Disorder in Children

302.85 Gender Identity Disorder in Adolescents or Adults

Specify **if (for sexually mature individuals):**

Sexually Attracted to Males

Sexually Attracted to Females

Sexually Attracted to Both

Sexually Attracted to Neither

◆ Diagnostic criteria for Generalized Anxiety Disorder 300.02

A. Excessive anxiety and worry (apprehensive expectation), occurring more days than not for at least 6 months, about a number of events or activities (such as work or school performance).

B. The person finds it difficult to control the worry.

C. The anxiety and worry are associated with three (or more) of the following six symptoms (with at least some symptoms present for more days than not for the past 6 months). **Note:** Only one item is required in children.

(1) restlessness or feeling keyed up or on edge
(2) being easily fatigued
(3) difficulty concentrating or mind going blank
(4) irritability
(5) muscle tension
(6) sleep disturbance (difficulty falling or staying asleep, or restless unsatisfying sleep)

D. The focus of the anxiety and worry is not confined to features of another clinical disorder, e.g., the anxiety or worry is not about having a panic attack (as in panic disorder), being embarrassed in public (as in social phobia), being contaminated (as in obsessive-compulsive disorder), being away from home or close relatives (as in separation anxiety disorder), gaining weight (as in anorexia nervosa), having multiple physical complaints (as in somatization disorder), or having a serious illness (as in hypochondriasis), and the anxiety and worry do not occur exclusively during post- traumatic stress disorder.

E. The anxiety, worry, or physical symptoms cause clinically significant distress or impairment in social, occupational, or other important areas of functioning.

F. The disturbance is not due to the direct physiological effects of a substance (e.g., a drug or abuse, a medication) or a general medical condition (e.g., hyperthyroidism) and does not occur exclusively during a mood disorder, a psychotic disorder, or a pervasive developmental disorder.

◆ Diagnostic criteria for Hypochondriasis 300.7

A. Preoccupation with fears of having, or the idea that one has, a serious disease based on the person's misinterpretation of bodily symptoms.

B. The preoccupation persists despite appropriate medical evaluation and reassurance.

C. The belief in criterion A is not of delusional intensity (as in delusional disorder, somatic type) and is not restricted to a circumscribed concern about appearance (as in body dysmorphic disorder).

D. The preoccupation causes clinically significant distress or impairment in social, occupational, or other important areas of functioning.

E. The duration of the disturbance is at least 6 months.

F. The preoccupation is not better accounted for by generalized anxiety disorder, obsessive-compulsive disorder, panic disorder, a major depressive episode, separation anxiety, or another somatoform disorder.

Specify if:

With Poor Insight: if, for most of the time during the current episode, the person does not recognize that the concern about having a serious illness is excessive or unreasonable

◆ Diagnostic criteria for Learning Disorder, Not Otherwise Specified 315.9

This category is for disorders in learning that do not meet criteria for any specific learning disorder. This category might include problems in all three areas (reading, mathematics, written expression) that together significantly interfere with academic achievement even though performance on tests measuring each individual skill is not substantially below that expected given the person's chronological age, measured intelligence, and age-appropriate education.

◆ Diagnostic criteria for Major Depressive Episode

A. Five (or more) of the following symptoms have been present during the same 2-week period and represent a change from previous functioning; at least one of the symptoms is either (1) depressed mood or (2) loss of interest or pleasure.

Note: Do not include symptoms that are clearly due to a general medical condition, or mood-incongruent delusions or hallucinations.

(1) depressed mood most of the day, nearly every day, as indicated by either subjective report (e.g., feels sad or empty) or observation made by others (e.g., appears tearful). **Note:** In children and adolescents, can be irritable mood.

(2) markedly diminished interest or pleasure in all, or almost all, activities most of the day, nearly every day (as indicated by either subjective account or observation made by others)

(3) significant weight loss when not dieting or weight gain (e.g., a change of more than 5% of body weight in a month), or decrease or increase in appetite nearly every day. **Note:** In children, consider failure to make expected weight gains.

(4) insomnia or hypersomnia nearly every day

(5) psychomotor agitation or retardation nearly every day (observable by others, not merely subjective feelings of restlessness or being slowed down)

(6) fatigue or loss of energy nearly every day

(7) feelings of worthlessness or excessive or inappropriate guilt (which may be delusional) nearly every day (not merely self-reproach or guilt about being sick)

(8) diminished ability to think or concentrate, or indecisiveness, nearly every day (either by subjective account or as observed by others)

(9) recurrent thoughts of death (not just fear of dying), recurrent suicidal ideation without a specific plan, or a suicide attempt or a specific plan for committing suicide

B. The symptoms do not meet criteria for a mixed episode.

C. The symptoms cause clinically significant distress or impairment in social, occupational, or other important areas of functioning.

D. The symptoms are not due to the direct physiological effects of a substance (e.g., a drug of abuse, a medication) or a general medical condition (e.g., hypothyroidism).

E. The symptoms are not better accounted for by bereavement, i.e., after the loss of a loved one, the symptoms persist for longer than 2 months or are characterized by marked functional impairment, morbid preoccupation with worthlessness, suicidal ideation, psychotic symptoms, or psycho-motor retardation.

◆ Diagnostic criteria for Major Depressive Disorder, Single Episode 296.2x

A. Presence of a single major depressive episode.

B. The major depressive episode is not better accounted for by schizoaffective disorder and is not superimposed on schizophrenia, schizophreniform disorder, delusional disorder, or psychotic disorder not otherwise specified.

C. There has never been a manic episode, a mixed episode, or a hypomanic episode.
Note: This exclusion does not apply if all of the manic-like, mixed-like, or hypomanic-like episodes are substance or treatment induced or are due to the direct physiological effects of a general medical condition.

Specify (for current or most recent episode):
Severity/Psychotic/Remission Specifiers
296.26 In full remission
296.25 In partial remission
296.21 Mild
296.22 Moderate
296.23 Severe Without Psychotic Features
296.24 Severe With Psychotic Features
296.20 Unspecified

◆ Diagnostic criteria for Major Depressive Disorder, Recurrent 296.3x

A. Presence of two or more major depressive episodes. **Note:** To be considered separate episodes, there must be an interval of at least 2 consecutive months in which criteria are not met for a major depressive episode.

B. The major depressive episodes are not better accounted for by schizoaffective disorder and are not superimposed on schizophrenia, schizophreniform disorder, delusional disorder, or psychotic disorder, not otherwise specified.

C. There has never been a manic episode, a mixed episode, or a hypomanic episode.
Note: This exclusion does not apply if all of the manic-like, mixed-like, or hypomanic-like episodes are substance or treatment induced or are due to the indirect physiological effects of a general medical condition.

Specify (for current or most recent episode):

Severity/Psychotic/Remission Specifiers

296.36 In full remission

296.35 In partial remission

296.31 Mild

296.32 Moderate

296.33 Severe Without Psychotic Features

296.34 Severe With Psychotic Features

296.30 Unspecified

◆ Diagnostic criteria for Mathematics Disorder 315.1 (see Academic Skills cluster, p 69).

◆ Diagnostic criteria for Mental Retardation 317, 318.x, 319 (see Cognitive/Adaptive Skills, Mental Retardation, p 61)

◆ Diagnostic criteria for Mixed Receptive-Expressive Language Disorder 315.32 (see Speech and Language cluster, p 83).

◆ Diagnostic criteria for Narcolepsy 347

A. Irresistible attacks of refreshing sleep that occur daily over at least 3 months.

B. The presence of one or both of the following:
   (1) cataplexy, (i.e., brief episodes of sudden bilateral loss of muscle tone, most often in association with intense emotion)
   (2) recurrent intrusions of elements of rapid eye movement (REM) sleep into the transition between sleep and wakefulness, as manifested by either hypnopompic or hypnagogic hallucinations or sleep paralysis at the beginning or end of sleep episodes

C. The disturbance is not due to the direct physiological effects of a substance (e.g., a drug of abuse, a medication) or another general medical condition.

◆ Diagnostic criteria for Nightmare Disorder 307.47

A. Repeated awakenings from the major sleep period or naps with detailed recall of extended and extremely frightening dreams, usually involving threats to survival, security, or self-esteem. The awakenings generally occur during the second half of the sleep period.

B. On awakening from the frightening dreams, the person rapidly becomes oriented and alert (in contrast to the confusion and disorientation seen in sleep terror disorder and some forms of epilepsy).

C. The dream experience, or the sleep disturbance resulting from the awakening, causes clinically significant distress or impairment in social, occupational, or other important areas of functioning.

D. The nightmares do not occur exclusively during the course of another mental disorder (e.g., a delirium, posttraumatic stress disorder), and are not due to the direct physiological effects of a substance (e.g., a drug of abuse, a medication), or a general medical condition.

◆ Diagnostic criteria for Not Otherwise Specified Categories (see specific category for code)

Because of the diversity of clinical presentations, it is impossible for the diagnostic nomenclature to cover every possible situation. For this reason, each diagnostic class has at least one Not Otherwise Specified (NOS) category and some classes have several NOS categories. There are four situations in which an NOS diagnosis may be appropriate:

- The presentation conforms to the general guidelines for a mental disorder in the diagnostic class, but the symptomatic picture does not meet the criteria for any of the specific disorders. This would occur either when the symptoms are below the diagnostic threshold for one of the specific disorders or when there is an atypical or mixed presentation.

- The presentation conforms to a symptom patterns that has not been included in the DSM-IV Classification but that causes clinically significant distress or impairment.

- There is uncertainty about etiology (i.e., whether the disorder is due to a general medical condition, is substance induced, or is primary).

- There is insufficient opportunity for complete data collection (e.g., in emergency situations) or inconsistent or contradictory information, but there is enough information to place it within a particular diagnostic class (e.g., the clinician determines that the individual has psychotic symptoms but does not have enough information to diagnose a specific psychotic disorder).

◆ Diagnostic criteria for Obsessive-Compulsive Disorder 300.3

A. Either obsessions or compulsions:

Obsessions as defined by (1), (2), (3), and (4):
(1) recurrent and persistent thoughts, impulses, or images that are experienced, at some time during the disturbance, as intrusive and inappropriate and that cause marked anxiety or distress
(2) the thoughts, impulses, or images are not simply excessive worries about real-life problems

(3) the person attempts to ignore or suppress such thoughts, impulses, or images, or to neutralize them with some other thought or action

(4) the person recognizes that the obsessional thoughts, impulses, or images are a product of his or her own mind (not imposed from without as in thought insertion)

Compulsions as defined by (1) and (2):

(1) repetitive behaviors (e.g., hand washing, ordering, checking) or mental acts (e.g., praying, counting, repeating words silently) that the person feels driven to perform in response to an obsession, or according to rules that must be applied rigidly

(2) the behaviors or mental acts are aimed at preventing or reducing distress or preventing some dreaded event or situation; however, these behaviors or mental acts either are not connected in a realistic way with what they are designed to neutralize or prevent or are clearly excessive

B. At some point during the course of the disorder, the person has recognized that the obsessions or compulsions are excessive or unreasonable. **Note:** This does not apply to children.

C. The obsessions or compulsions cause marked distress, are time consuming (take more than 1 hour a day), or significantly interfere with the person's normal routine, occupational (or academic) functioning, or usual social activities or relationships.

D. If another clinical disorder is present, the content of the obsessions or compulsions is not restricted to it (e.g., preoccupation with food in the presence of an eating disorder; hair pulling in the presence of body dysmorphic disorder; preoccupation with drugs in the presence of a substance use disorder; preoccupation with having a serious illness in the presence of hypochondriasis; preoccupation with sexual urges or fantasies in the presence of a paraphilia; or guilty ruminations in the presence of major depressive disorder).

E. The disturbance is not due to the direct physiological effects of a substance (e.g., a drug of abuse, a medication), or a general medical condition.

Specify **if:**

With Poor Insight: if, for most of the time during the current episode, the person does not recognize that the obsessions and compulsions are excessive or unreasonable.

◆ Diagnostic criteria for Oppositional Defiant Disorder 313.81

A. A pattern of negativistic, hostile, and defiant behavior lasting at least 6 months, during which four (or more) of the following are present:

(1) often loses temper

(2) often argues with adults

(3) often actively defies or refuses to comply with adults' requests or rules

(4) often deliberately annoys people

(5) often blames others for his or her mistakes or misbehavior

(6) is often touchy or easily annoyed by others

(7) is often angry and resentful

(8) is often spiteful or vindictive

Note: Consider a criterion met only if the behavior occurs more frequently than is typically observed in individuals of comparable age and developmental level.

B. The disturbance in behavior causes clinically significant impairment in social, academic, or occupational functioning.

C. The behaviors do not occur exclusively during the course of a psychotic or mood disorder.

D. Criteria are not met for conduct disorder, and, if the individual is age 18 years or older, criteria are not met for antisocial personality disorder.

◆ Diagnostic criteria for Pain Disorder 307.80

A. Pain in one or more anatomical sites is the predominant focus of the clinical presentation and is of sufficient severity to warrant clinical attention.

B. The pain causes clinically significant distress or impairment in social, occupational, or other important areas of functioning.

C. Psychological factors are judged to have an important role in the onset, severity, exacerbation, or maintenance of the pain.

D. The symptom or deficit is not intentionally produced or feigned (as in factitious disorder or malingering).

E. The pain is not better accounted for by a mood, anxiety, or psychotic disorder, and does not meet criteria for dyspareunia.

Specify if:

Acute: duration of less than 6 months

Chronic: duration of 6 months or longer

307.89 Pain Disorder Associated With Both Psychological Factors and a General Medical Condition: both psychological factors and a general medical condition are judged to have important roles in the onset, severity, exacerbation, or maintenance of the pain. The associated general medical condition or anatomical site of the pain (see below) is coded.

Specify if:

Acute: duration of less than 6 months

Chronic: duration of 6 months or longer

Note: The following is not considered to be a mental disorder and is included here to facilitate differential diagnosis.

Pain Disorder Associated With a General Medical Condition: a general medical condition has a major role in the onset, severity, exacerbation, or maintenance of the pain. (If psychological factors are present, they are not judged to have a major role in the onset, severity, exacerbation, or maintenance of the pain.) The diagnostic code for the pain is selected based on the associated general medical condition if one has been established or on the anatomical location of the pain if the underlying general medical condition is not yet clearly established—for example, low back (**724.2**), sciatic (**724.3**), pelvic (**625.9**), headache (**784.0**), facial (**784.0**), chest (**786.50**), joint (**719.4**), bone (**733.90**), abdominal (**789.0**), breast (**611.71**), renal (**788.0**), eye (**379.91**), throat (**784.1**), tooth (**525.9**), and urinary (**788.0**).

◆ Diagnostic criteria for Panic Disorder With Agoraphobia 300.21

A. Both (1) and (2):
   (1) recurrent unexpected panic attacks
   (2) at least one of the attacks has been followed by 1 month (or more) of one (or more) of the following:
      (a) persistent concern about having additional attacks
      (b) worry about the implications of the attack or its consequences (e.g., losing control, having a heart attack, "going crazy")
      (c) a significant change in behavior related to the attacks
B. The presence of agoraphobia.
C. The panic attacks are not due to the direct physiological effects of a substance (e.g., a drug of abuse, a medication) or a general medical condition (e.g., hyperthyroidism).
D. The panic attacks are not better accounted for by another mental disorder such as social phobia (e.g., occurring on exposure to feared social situations), specific phobia (e.g., on exposure to a specific phobic situation), obsessive-compulsive disorder (e.g., on exposure to dirt in someone with an obsession about contamination), posttraumatic stress disorder (e.g., in response to stimuli associated with a severe stressor), or separation anxiety disorder (e.g., in response to being away from home or close relatives).

◆ Diagnostic criteria for Panic Disorder Without Agoraphobia 300.01

A. Both (1) and (2):
   (1) recurrent unexpected panic attacks
   (2) at least one of the attacks has been followed by 1 month (or more) of one (or more) of the following:
      (a) persistent concern about having additional attacks
      (b) worry about the implications of the attack or its consequences (e.g., losing control, having a heart attack, "going crazy")
      (c) a significant change in behavior related to the attacks

B. Absence of agoraphobia.

C. The panic attacks are not due to the direct physiological effects of a substance (e.g., a drug of abuse, a medication) or a general medical condition (e.g., hyperthyroidism).

D. The panic attacks are not better accounted for by another mental disorder such as social phobia (e.g., occurring on exposure to feared social situations), specific phobia (e.g., on exposure to a specific phobic situation), obsessive-compulsive disorder (e.g., on exposure to dirt in someone with an obsession about contamination), posttraumatic stress disorder (e.g., in response to stimuli associated with a severe stressor), or separation anxiety disorder (e.g., in response to being away from home or close relatives).

◆ Diagnostic criteria for Parasomnia, Not Otherwise Specified 307.47

The Parasomnia, Not Otherwise Specified category is for disturbances that are characterized by abnormal behavioral or physiological events during sleep or sleep-wake transitions, but that do not meet criteria for a more specific parasomnia. Examples include:

(1) REM sleep behavior disorder: motor activity, often of a violent nature, that arises during rapid eye movement (REM) sleep. Unlike sleepwalking, these episodes tend to occur later in the night and are associated with vivid dream recall.

(2) Sleep paralysis: an inability to perform voluntary movement during the transition between wakefulness and sleep. The episodes may occur at sleep onset (hypnagogic) or with awakening (hypnopompic). The episodes are usually associated with extreme anxiety and, in some cases, fear of impending death. Sleep paralysis occurs commonly as an ancillary symptom of narcolepsy and, in such cases, should not be coded separately.

(3) Situations in which the clinician has concluded that a parasomnia is present but is unable to determine whether it is primary, due to a general medical condition, or substance induced.

◆ Diagnostic criteria for Phonological Disorder 315.39 (see Speech and Language cluster, p 83).

◆ Diagnostic criteria for Pica 307.52

A. Persistent eating of nonnutritive substances for a period of at least 1 month.

B. The eating of nonnutritive substance is inappropriate to the developmental level.

C. The eating behavior is not part of a culturally sanctioned practice.

D. If the eating behavior occurs exclusively during the course of another mental disorder (e.g., mental retardation, pervasive developmental disorder, schizophrenia), it is sufficiently severe to warrant independent clinical attention.

◆ Diagnostic criteria for Posttraumatic Stress Disorder 309.81

A. The person has been exposed to a traumatic event in which both of the following were present:

    (1) the person experienced, witnessed, or was confronted with an event or events that involved actual or threatened death or serious injury, or a threat to the physical integrity of self or others

    (2) the person's response involved intense fear, helplessness, or horror. **Note:** In children, this may be expressed instead by disorganized or agitated behavior.

B. The traumatic event is persistently reexperienced in one (or more) of the following ways:

    (1) recurrent and intrusive distressing recollections of the event, including images, thoughts, or perceptions. **Note:** In young children, repetitive play may occur in themes or aspects of the trauma are expressed.

    (2) recurrent distressing dreams of the event. **Note:** In children, there may be frightening dreams without recognizable content.

    (3) acting or feeling as if the traumatic event were recurring (includes a sense of reliving the experience, illusions, hallucinations, and dissociative flashback episodes, including those that occur on awakening or when intoxicated. **Note:** In young children, trauma-specific reenactment may occur.

    (4) intense psychological distress at exposure to internal or external cues that symbolize or resemble an aspect of the traumatic event

C. Persistent avoidance of stimuli associated with the trauma and numbing of general responsiveness (not present before the trauma) as indicated by three (or more) of the following:

    (1) efforts to avoid thoughts, feelings, or conversations associated with the trauma

    (2) efforts to avoid activities, places, or people that arouse recollections of the trauma

    (3) inability to recall an important aspect of the trauma

    (4) markedly diminished interest or participation in significant activities

    (5) feeling of detachment or estrangement from others

    (6) restricted range of affect (e.g., unable to have loving feelings)

    (7) sense of a foreshortened future (e.g., does not expect to have a career, marriage, children, or a normal life span)

D. Persistent symptoms of increased arousal (not present before the trauma), as indicated by two (or more) of the following:

    (1) difficulty falling or staying asleep

    (2) irritability or outbursts of anger

    (3) difficulty concentrating

    (4) hypervigilance

    (5) exaggerated startle response

E. Duration of the disturbance (symptoms in criteria B, C, and D) is more than 1 month.

F. The disturbance causes clinically significant distress or impairment in social, occupational, or other important areas of functioning.

Specify if:

Acute: if duration of symptoms is less than 3 months

Chronic: if duration of symptoms is 3 months or more

Specify if:

With Delayed Onset: if onset of symptoms is at least 6 months after the stressor

◆ Diagnostic criteria for Primary Hypersomnia 307.44

A. The predominant complaint is excessive sleepiness for at least 1 month (or less if recurrent) as evidenced by either prolonged sleep episodes or daytime sleep episodes that occur almost daily.

B. The excessive sleepiness causes clinically significant distress or impairment in social, occupational, or other important areas of functioning.

C. The excessive sleepiness is not better accounted for by insomnia and does not occur exclusively during the course of another sleep disorder (e.g., narcolepsy, breathing-related sleep disorder, circadian rhythm sleep disorder, or a parasomnia) and cannot be accounted for by an inadequate amount of sleep.

D. The disturbance does not occur exclusively during the course of another mental disorder.

E. The disturbance is not due to the direct physiological effects of a substance (e.g., a drug of abuse, a medication), or a general medical condition.

Specify if:

Recurrent: if there are periods of excessive sleepiness that last at least 3 days occurring several times a year for at least 2 years

◆ Diagnostic criteria for Primary Insomnia 307.42

A. The predominant complaint is difficulty initiating or maintaining sleep, or nonrestorative sleep, for at least 1 month.

B. The sleep disturbance (or associated daytime fatigue) causes clinically significant distress or impairment in social, occupational, or other important areas of functioning.

C. The sleep disturbance does not occur exclusively during the course of narcolepsy, breathing-related sleep disorder, circadian rhythm sleep disorder, or a parasomnia.

D. The disturbance does not occur exclusively during the course of another mental disorder (e.g., major depressive disorder, generalized anxiety disorder, a delirium)

E. The disturbance is not due to the direct physiological effects of a substance (e.g., a drug of abuse, a medication), or a general medical condition.

◆ Diagnostic criteria for Reading Disorder 315.00 (see Academic Skills cluster, p 69).

◆ Diagnostic criteria for Rett's Disorder 299.80

A. All of the following:
   (1) apparently normal prenatal and perinatal development
   (2) apparently normal psychomotor development through the first 5 months after birth
   (3) normal head circumference at birth
B. Onset of all of the following after the period of normal development:
   (1) deceleration of head growth between ages 5 and 48 months
   (2) loss of previously acquired purposeful hand skills between ages 5 and 30 months with the subsequent development of stereotyped hand movements (i.e., hand-wringing or hand washing)
   (3) loss of social engagement early in the course (although often social interaction develops later)
   (4) appearance of poorly coordinated gait or trunk movements
   (5) severely impaired expressive and receptive language development with severe psychomotor retardation

◆ Diagnostic criteria for Rumination Disorder 307.53

A. Repeated regurgitation and rechewing of food for a period of at least 1 month following a period of normal functioning.
B. The behavior is not due to an associated gastrointestinal or other general medical condition (e.g., esophageal reflux).
C. The behavior does not occur exclusively during the course of anorexia nervosa or bulimia nervosa. If the symptoms occur exclusively during the course of mental retardation or a pervasive developmental disorder, they are sufficiently severe to warrant independent clinical attention.

◆ Diagnostic criteria for Separation Anxiety Disorder 309.21

A. Developmentally inappropriate and excessive anxiety concerning separation from home or from those to whom the individual is attached, as evidenced by three (or more) of the following:

(1) recurrent excessive distress when separation from home or major attachment figures occurs or is anticipated

(2) persistent and excessive worry about losing, or about possible harm befalling, major attachment figures

(3) persistent and excessive worry that an untoward event will lead to separation from a major attachment figure (e.g., getting lost or being kidnapped)

(4) persistent reluctance or refusal to go to school or elsewhere because of fear of separation

(5) persistently and excessively fearful or reluctant to be alone or without major attachment figures at home or without significant adults in other settings

(6) persistent reluctance or refusal to go to sleep without being near a major attachment figure or to sleep away from home

(7) repeated nightmares involving the theme of separation

(8) repeated complaints of physical symptoms (such as headaches, stomachaches, nausea, or vomiting) when separation from major attachment figures occurs or is anticipated

B. The duration of the disturbance is at least 4 weeks.

C. The onset is before age 18 years.

D. The disturbance causes clinically significant distress or impairment in social, academic (occupational), or other important areas of functioning.

E. The disturbance does not occur exclusively during the course of a pervasive developmental disorder, schizophrenia, or other psychotic disorder and, in adolescents and adults, is not better accounted for by panic disorder with agoraphobia.

Specify if:

Early Onset: if onset occurs before age 6 years

◆ Diagnostic criteria for Sleep Terror Disorder 307.46

A. Recurrent episodes of abrupt awakening from sleep, usually occurring during the first third of the major sleep episode, and beginning with a panicky scream.

B. Intense fear and signs of autonomic arousal, such as tachycardia, rapid breathing, and sweating, during each episode.

C. Relative unresponsiveness to efforts of others to comfort the person during the episode.

D. No detailed dream is recalled and there is amnesia for the episode.

E. The episodes cause clinically significant distress or impairment in social, occupational, or other important areas of functioning.

F. The disturbance is not due to the direct physiological effects of a substance (e.g., a drug of abuse, a medication), or a general medical condition.

◆ Diagnostic criteria for Sleepwalking Disorder 307.46

A. Repeated episodes of rising from bed during sleep and walking about, usually occurring during the first third of the major sleep episode.

B. While sleepwalking, the person has a blank, staring face, is relatively unresponsive to the efforts of others to communicate with him or her, and can be awakened only with great difficulty.

C. On awakening (either from the sleepwalking episode or the next morning), the person has amnesia for the episode.

D. Within several minutes after awakening from the sleepwalking episode, there is no impairment of mental activity or behavior (although there may initially be a short period of confusion or disorientation).

E. The sleepwalking causes clinically significant distress or impairment in social, occupational, or other important areas of functioning.

F. The disturbance is not due to the direct physiological effects of a substance (e.g., a drug of abuse, a medication), or a general medical condition.

◆ Diagnostic criteria for Social Phobia 300.23

A. A marked and persistent fear of one or more social or performance situations in which the person is exposed to unfamiliar people or to possible scrutiny by others. The individual fears that he or she will act in a way (or show anxiety symptoms) that will be humiliating or embarrassing. **Note:** In children, there must be evidence of the capacity for age-appropriate social relationships with familiar people and the anxiety must occur in peer settings, not just in interactions with adults.

B. Exposure to the feared social situation almost invariably provokes anxiety, which may take the form of a situationally bound or situationally predisposed panic attack. **Note:** In children, the anxiety may be expressed by crying, tantrums, freezing, or shrinking from social situations with unfamiliar people.

C. The person recognizes that the fear is excessive or unreasonable. **Note:** In children, this feature may be absent.

D. The feared social or performance situations are avoided or else are endured with intense anxiety or distress.

E. The avoidance, anxious anticipation, or distress in the feared social or performance situation(s) interferes significantly with the person's normal routine, occupational (academic) functioning, or social activities or relationships, or there is marked distress about having the phobia.

F. In individuals under age 18 years, the duration is at least 6 months.

G. The fear or avoidance is not due to the direct physiological effects of a substance (e.g., a drug of abuse, a medication) or a general medical condition and is not better accounted for by another mental disorder (e.g., panic disorder with or without agoraphobia, separation anxiety disorder, body dysmorphic disorder, a pervasive developmental disorder, or schizoid personality disorder).

H. If a general medical condition or another mental disorder is present, the fear in criterion A is unrelated to it, e.g., the fear is not of stuttering, trembling in Parkinson's disease, or exhibiting abnormal eating behavior in anorexia nervosa or bulimia nervosa.

Specify if:

Generalized: if the fears include most social situations (also consider the additional diagnosis of avoidant personality disorder)

◆ Diagnostic criteria for Somatization Disorder 300.82

A. A history of many physical complaints beginning before age 30 years that occur over a period of several years and result in treatment being sought or significant impairment in social, occupational, or other important areas of functioning.

B. Each of the following criteria must have been met, with individual symptoms occurring at any time during the course of the disturbance:

(1) *four pain symptoms:* a history of pain related to at least four different sites or functions (e.g., head, abdomen, back, joints, extremities, chest, rectum, during menstruation, during sexual intercourse, or during urination)

(2) *two gastrointestinal symptoms:* a history of at least two gastrointestinal symptoms other than pain (e.g., nausea, bloating, vomiting other than during pregnancy, diarrhea, or intolerance of several different foods)

(3) *one sexual symptom:* a history of at least one sexual or reproductive symptom other than pain (e.g., sexual indifference, erectile, or ejaculatory dysfunction, irregular menses, excessive menstrual bleeding, vomiting throughout pregnancy)

(4) *one pseudoneurological symptom:* a history of at least one symptom or deficit suggesting a neurological condition not limited to pain (conversion symptoms such as impaired coordination or balance, paralysis or localized weakness, difficulty swallowing or lump in throat, aphonia, urinary retention, hallucinations, loss of touch or pain sensation, double vision, blindness, deafness, seizures; dissociative symptoms such as amnesia; or loss of consciousness other than fainting)

C. Either (1) or (2):

(1) after appropriate investigation, each of the symptoms in criterion B cannot be fully explained by a known general medical condition or the direct effects of a substance (e.g., a drug of abuse, a medication)

(2) when there is a related general medical condition, the physical complaints or resulting social or occupational impairment are in excess of what would be expected from the history, physical examination, or laboratory findings

D. The symptoms are not intentionally produced or feigned (as in factitious disorder or malingering).

◆ Diagnostic criteria for Somatoform Disorder, Not Otherwise Specified 300.82

This category includes disorders with somatoform symptoms that do not meet the criteria for any specific somatoform disorder. Examples include:

(1) Pseudocyesis: a false belief of being pregnant that is associated with objective signs of pregnancy, which may include abdominal enlargement (although the umbilicus does not become everted), reduced menstrual flow, amenorrhea, subjective sensation of fetal movement, nausea, breast engorgement and secretions, and labor pains at the expected date of delivery. Endocrine changes may be present, but the syndrome cannot be explained by a general medical condition that causes endocrine changes (e.g., a hormone-secreting tumor).

(2) A disorder involving nonpsychotic hypochondriacal symptoms of less than 6 month's duration

(3) A disorder involving unexplained physical complaints (e.g., fatigue or body weakness) of less than 6 months' duration that are not due to another mental disorder.

◆ Diagnostic criteria for Specific Phobia 300.29

A. Marked and persistent feat that is excessive or unreasonable, cued by the presence or anticipation of a specific object or situation (e.g., flying, heights, animals, receiving an injection, seeing blood).

B. Exposure to the phobic stimulus almost invariably provokes an immediate anxiety response, which may take the form of a situationally bound or situationally predisposed panic attack. **Note:** In children, the anxiety may be expressed by crying, tantrums, freezing, or clinging.

C. The person recognizes that the fear is excessive or unreasonable. **Note:** In children, this feature may be absent.

D. The phobic situation(s) is avoided or else is endured with intense anxiety or distress.

E. The avoidance, anxious anticipation, or distress in the feared situation(s) interferes significantly with the person's normal routine, occupational (or academic) functioning, or social activities or relationships, or there is marked distress about having the phobia.

F. In individuals under age 18 years, the duration is at least 6 months.

G. The anxiety, panic attacks, or phobic avoidance associated with the specific object or situation are not better accounted for by another mental disorder, such as obsessive-compulsive disorder (e.g., fear of dirt in someone with an obsession about contamination), posttraumatic stress disorder, (e.g., avoidance of stimuli associated with a severe stressor), separation anxiety disorder (e.g., avoidance of school), social phobia (e.g., avoidance of social situations because of fear of embarrassment), panic disorder with agoraphobia, or agoraphobia without history of panic disorder.

Specify type:

Animal type

Natural Environment Type (e.g., heights, storms, water)

Blood-Injection-Injury Type

Situational Type: (e.g., airplanes, elevators, enclosed places)

Other Type: (e.g., phobic avoidance of situations that may lead to choking, vomiting, or contracting an illness; in children, avoidance of loud sounds or costumed characters)

◆ (Specified Psychological Factor) Affecting…(*Indicate the General Medical Condition*) 316

A. A general medical condition is present.

B. Psychological factors adversely affect the general medical condition in one of the following ways:

    (1) the factors have influenced the course of the general medical condition as shown by a close temporal association between the psychological factors and the development or exacerbation of, or delayed recovery from, the general medical condition

    (2) the factors interfere with the treatment of the general medical condition

    (3) the factors constitute additional health risks for the individual

    (4) stress-related physiological responses precipitate or exacerbate symptoms of the general medical condition

Choose name based on the nature of the psychological factors (if more than one factor is present, indicate the most prominent):

Mental Disorder Affecting…*[Indicate the General Medical Condition]* (e.g., a clinical disorder such as Major Depressive disorder delaying recovery from a myocardial infarction)

Psychological Symptoms Affecting…*[Indicate the General Medical Condition]* (e.g., depressive symptoms delaying recovery from surgery; anxiety exacerbating asthma)

Personality Traits or Coping Style Affecting…*[Indicate the General Medical Condition]* (e.g., pathological denial of the need for surgery in a patient with cancer; hostile, pressured behavior contributing to cardiovascular disease)

Maladaptive Health Behaviors Affecting... *[Indicate the General Medical Condition]* (e.g., overeating, lack of exercise, unsafe sex)

Stress-Related Physiological Response Affecting... *[Indicate the General Medical Condition]* (e.g., stress-related exacerbations of ulcer, hypertension, arrhythmia, or tension headache)

Other or Unspecified Psychological Factors Affecting... *[Indicate the General Medical Condition]* (e.g., interpersonal, cultural, or religious factors)

◆ Diagnostic criteria for Stereotypic Movement Disorder 307.3

A. Repetitive, seemingly driven, and nonfunctional motor behavior (e.g., hand shaking or waving, body rocking, head banging, mouthing of objects, self-biting, picking at skin or bodily orifices, hitting own body).

B. The behavior markedly interferes with normal activities or results in self-inflicted bodily injury that requires medical treatment (or would result in an injury if preventive measures were not used).

C. If mental retardation is present, the stereotypic or self-injurious behavior is of sufficient severity to become a focus of treatment.

D. The behavior is not better accounted for by a compulsion (as in obsessive-compulsive disorder), a tic (as in tic disorder), a stereotypy that is part of a pervasive developmental disorder, or hair pulling (as in trichotillomania).

E. The behavior is not due to the direct physiological effects of a substance or a general medical condition.

F. The behavior persist for 4 weeks or longer.

Specify if:

With Self-Injurious Behavior: if the behavior results in bodily damage that requires specific treatment (or that would result in bodily damage if protective measures were not used)

◆ Diagnostic criteria for Stuttering 307.0 (see Speech and Language cluster, p 83).

◆ Criteria for Substance Abuse 305

A. A maladaptive pattern of substance use leading to clinically significant impairment or distress, as manifested by one (or more) of the following, occurring within a 12-month period:

(1) recurrent substance use resulting in a failure to fulfill major role obligations at work, school, or home (e.g., repeated absences or poor work performance related to substance use; substance-related absences, suspensions, or expulsions from school; neglect of children or household)

(2) recurrent substance use in situations in which it is physically hazardous (e.g., driving an automobile or operating a machine when impaired by substance use)

(3) recurrent substance-related problems (e.g., arrests for substance-related disorderly conduct)

(4) continued substance use despite having persistent or recurrent social or interpersonal problems caused or exacerbated by the effects of the substance (e.g., arguments with spouse about consequences of intoxication, physical fights)

B. The symptoms have never met the criteria for substance dependence for this class of substance.

◆ Criteria for Substance Dependence 305

A maladaptive pattern of substance use, leading to clinically significant impairment or distress, as manifested by three (or more) of the following:

(1) tolerance, as defined by either of the following:

    (a) a need for markedly increased amounts of the substance to achieve intoxication or desired effect

    (b) markedly diminished effect with continued use of the same amount of the substance

(2) withdrawal, as manifested by either of the following:

    (a) the characteristic withdrawal syndrome for the substance (refer to criteria A and B of the criteria sets for withdrawal from the specific substances)

    (b) the same (or a closely related) substance is taken to relieve or avoid withdrawal symptoms

(3) the substance is often taken in larger amounts or over a longer period than was intended

(4) there is a persistent desire or unsuccessful efforts to cut down or control substance use

(5) a great deal of time is spent in activities necessary to obtain the substance (e.g., visiting multiple doctors or driving long distances), use the substance (e.g., chain-smoking), or recover from its effects

(6) important social, occupational, or recreational activities are given up or reduced because of substance use

(7) the substance use is continued despite knowledge of having a persistent or recurrent physical or psychological problem that is likely to have been caused or exacerbated by the substance (e.g., current cocaine use despite recognition of cocaine-induced depression, or continued drinking despite recognition that an ulcer was made worse by alcohol consumption)

Specify if:

With Physiological Dependence: evidence of tolerance or withdrawal (i.e., either from item 1 or 2 is present)

Without Physiological Dependence: no evidence of tolerance or withdrawal (i.e., neither item 1 nor 2 is present)

Course specifiers (see text for definitions):

Early Full Remission
Early Partial Remission
Sustained Full Remission
Sustained Partial Remission
On Agonist Therapy
In a Controlled Environment

◆ Criteria for Substance Intoxication 305

A. The development of a reversible substance-specific syndrome due to recent ingestion of (or exposure to) a substance. **Note:** Different substances may produce similar or identical syndromes.

B. Clinically significant maladaptive behavioral or psychological changes that are due to the effect of the substance on the central nervous system (e.g., belligerence, mood lability, cognitive impairment, impaired judgment, impaired social or occupational functioning) and develop during or shortly after use of the substance.

C. The symptoms are not due to a general medical condition and are not better accounted for by another mental disorder.

◆ Criteria for Substance Withdrawal 292.0

A. The development of a substance-specific syndrome due to the cessation of (or reduction in) substance use that has been heavy and prolonged.

B. The substance-specific syndrome causes clinically significant distress or impairment in social, occupational, or other important areas of functioning.

C. The symptoms are not due to a general medical condition and are not better accounted for by another mental disorder.

◆ Codes for Specific Substances

303.00 Alcohol Intoxication
303.90 Alcohol Dependence
304.00 Opioid Dependence
304.10 Sedative, Hypnotic, or Anxiolytic Dependence
304.20 Cocaine Dependence
304.30 Cannabis Dependence
304.40 Amphetamine Dependence
304.50 Hallucinogen Dependence
304.60 Inhalant Dependence
304.90 Other (or Unknown) Substance Dependence

304.90 Phencyclidine Dependence

305.00 Alcohol Abuse

305.10 Nicotine Dependence

305.20 Cannabis Abuse

305.30 Hallucinogen Abuse

305.40 Sedative, Hypnotic, or Anxiolytic Abuse

305.50 Opioid Abuse

305.60 Cocaine Abuse

305.70 Amphetamine Abuse

305.90 Caffeine Intoxication

305.90 Inhalant Abuse

305.90 Other (or Unknown) Substance Abuse

305.90 Phencyclidine Abuse

◆ Diagnostic criteria for Tourette's Disorder 307.23 (see Repetitive Behavioral cluster, p 269).

◆ Diagnostic criteria for Transient Tic Disorder 307.21 (see Repetitive Behavioral Patterns cluster, p 269).

◆ Diagnostic criteria for Trichotillomania 312.39

A. Recurrent pulling out of one's hair resulting in noticeable hair loss.

B. An increasing sense of tension immediately before pulling out the hair or when attempting to resist the behavior.

C. Pleasure, gratification, or relief when pulling out the hair.

D. The disturbance is not better accounted for by another mental disorder and is not due to a general medical condition (e.g., a dermatological condition).

E. The disturbance causes clinically significant distress or impairment in social, occupational, or other important areas of functioning.

◆ Diagnostic criteria for Undifferentiated Somatoform Disorder 300.82

A. One or more physical complaints (e.g., fatigue, loss of appetite, gastrointestinal or urinary complaints).

B. Either (1) or (2):

    (1) after appropriate investigation, the symptoms cannot be fully explained by a known general medical condition or the direct effects of a substance (e.g., a drug of abuse, a medication)

(2) when there is a related general medical condition, the physical complaints or resulting social or occupational impairment is in excess of what would be expected from the history, physical examination, or laboratory findings

C. The symptoms cause clinically significant distress or impairment in social, occupational, or other important areas of functioning.

D. The duration of the disturbance is at least 6 months.

E. The disturbance is not better accounted for by another mental disorder (e.g., another somatoform disorder, sexual dysfunction, mood disorder, anxiety disorder, sleep disorder, or psychotic disorder).

F. The symptom is not intentionally produced or feigned (as in factitious disorder or malingering).

Appendix D

Reviewers

Richard R. Abidin, PhD, Curry Programs in Clinical and School Psychology, Charlottesville, VA

F. Jay Ach, MD, Premier Medical Associates, Cincinnati, OH

Jon R. Almquist, MD, Virginia Mason Clinic, Seattle, WA

Renner S. Anderson, MD, Park Nicollet Medical Foundation, Minneapolis, MN

Virginia Q. Anthony, American Academy of Child and Adolescent Psychiatry, Washington, DC

F. Daniel Armstrong, PhD, University of Miami School of Medicine, Miami, FL

Stephen Barnett, MD, University of Texas, Galveston, TX

Mark A. Barnhill, DO, Iowa Physicians Clinic, Des Moines, IA

Judith Ann Bays, MD, Emanuel Hospital, Portland, OR

Roberta Ann Beach, MD, Denver Health and Hospital, Denver, CO

Carl Bell, MD, Community Medical Health Center, Chicago, IL

Debra Bendell-Estroff, PhD, Department of Psychiatry, Kaiser Permanente, Fremont, CA

Marilyn B. Benoit, MD, American Academy of Child and Adolescent Psychiatry, Washington, DC

Catherine Beyer, MD, Major James H. Rumbaugh Child and Adolescent Mental Health Clinic, Fayetteville, NC

Boris Birmaher, MD, Western Psychiatric Institute Clinic, Pittsburgh, PA

William G. Bithoney, MD, Children's Hospital, Boston, MA

Robin Krause Blitz, MD, Prince George's Hospital Center, Bethesda, MD

William E. Boyle, Jr., MD, Dartmouth-Hitchcock Medical Center, Lebanon, NH

Susan J. Bradley, MD, Hospital for Sick Children, Ontario, Canada

David Bromberg, MD, FAAP, The Pediatric Center, Frederick, MD

Oscar Bukstein, MD, Western Psychiatric Institute and Clinics, Pittsburgh, PA

Regina Bussing, MD, University of Florida, Gainesville, FL

Magda Campbell, MD, New York University Medical Center, New York, NY

Dennis P. Cantwell, MD, University of California, Los Angeles, CA

David L. Chadwick, MD, Children's Hospital and Health Center, San Diego, CA

Edward R. Christophersen, POD, FAAP, Children's Mercy Hospital, Kansas City, MO

Susan Coates, PhD, CGIC Psychiatric Associates of Manhattan, P.C., New York, NY

George J. Cohen, MD, National Consortium for Child Mental Health Services, Rockville, MD

William Cohen, MD, Children's Hospital of Pittsburgh, Pittsburgh, PA

William Coleman, MD, University of North Carolina, Chapel Hill, NC

William Carl Cooley, MD, Dartmouth-Hitchcock Medical Center, Lebanon, NH

Daniel L. Coury, MD, Ohio State Medical Center, Columbus, OH

Edward O. Cox, MD, Butterworth Pediatric Clinics, Grand Rapids, MI

Margaret Cox, MD, Canadian Paediatrics Society, Ottawa, Canada

Carin Cunningham, PhD, Mt. Sinai Medical Center, Cleveland, OH

A. Todd Davis, MD, Children's Memorial Hospital, Chicago, IL

Anthony Dekker, DO, University of Health Sciences College of Osteopathic Medicine, Kansas City, MO

Martha Bridge Denckla, MD, The Kennedy Institute, Baltimore, MD

Jean Dorval, MD, Canadian Paediatric Society, Quebec, Canada

Mina Dulcan, MD, Children's Memorial Hospital, Chicago, IL

Dan Earl, DO, James H. Quillen College of Medicine, Family Medicine Associates, Johnson City, TN

Andrea J. Eberle, MD, PhD, University of Tennessee Medical Center at Knoxville, Knoxville, TN

Jean Elbert, MD, University of Oklahoma Child Study Center, Oklahoma City, OK

Glen Elliott, MD, Langley Porter Psychiatric Institute, San Francisco, CA

Gerald Erenberg, MD, Cleveland Clinic Children's Hospital, Cleveland, OH

Ann R. Ernst, PhD, Medical Associates Clinic, Dubuque, IA

Mary Evers-Szostak, PhD, Durham Pediatrics, PA, Durham, NC

Heidi Feldman, MD, Children's Hospital of Pittsburgh, Pittsburgh, PA

Richard Ferber, MD, Children's Hospital, Boston, MA

Al Finch, PhD, Citadel, SC

Martin Fisher, MD, North Shore University Hospital, Manhasset, NY

John Fontanesi, PhD, University of California at San Diego Medical Center, San Diego, CA

Joel Frader, MD, Children's Hospital of Pittsburgh, Pittsburgh, PA

Stanford B. Friedman, MD, Montefiore Medical Center, Bronx, NY

Barbara Geller, MD, Washington University School of Medicine, St. Louis, MO

Joan Gerring, MD, Kennedy Kreiger Institute, Baltimore, MD

Stephan Glicken, MD, New England Medical Center, Boston, MA

Stuart J. Goldman, MD, Children's Hospital, Boston, MA

Peter Gorski, MD, Massachusetts General Hospital, Boston, MA

Marvin Gottlieb, MD, Hackensack Medical Center, Hackensack, NJ

Estherann Grace, MD, Children's Hospital, Boston, MA

Mary Graham, American Academy of Child and Adolescent Psychiatry, Washington, DC

John Lewis Green, MD, Elmwood Pediatric Group, Rochester, NY

Morris Green, MD, Indiana University School of Medicine, Indianapolis, IN

Joseph Greensher, MD, Winthrop University Hospital, Mineola, NY

Stanley Greenspan, MD, National Center for Clinical Infant Programs, Washington, DC

Linda S. Grossman, MD, University of Maryland at Baltimore, Baltimore, MD

Julian Stuart Haber, MD, FAAP, Pediatrics, Ft. Worth, TX

Robert Haggerty, MD, University of Rochester School of Medicine, Rochester, NY

Robert E. Hannemann, MD, Arnett Clinic, Lafayette, IN

Robert Harmon, MD, University of Colorado, Denver, CO

Joan R. Hebeler, MD, University of Texas Medical Branch of Galveston, Galveston, TX

Viking A. Hedberg, MD, University of Rochester, Rochester, NY

Pamela D. Hogen, PsyD, Children's Hospital, Boston, MA

Ilene J. Holt, PhD, Children's Memorial Hospital, Chicago, IL

Stephen Houseworth, PhD, Rankin Clinical Research Unit, Durham, NC

Helene Rabena Hubbard, MD, PhD, Pediatric Private Practice, Hawkinsville, GA

Christine Hunter, MA, University of Minnesota, Minneapolis, MN

Linda K. Hurley, PhD, Fort Worth Pediatrics, Fort Worth, TX

Peter Jensen, MD, National Institute of Mental Health, Rockville, MD

Barbara Johnson, MD, Western Psychiatric Institute and Clinics, Pittsburgh, PA

Chet Johnson, MD, Klingberg Center for Child Development, Morgantown, WV

Robert Johnson, MD, New Jersey Medical Center, Newark, NJ

Lawrence Moral Jones, MD, FAAP, East Louisville Pediatrics, Louisville, KY

Kathy Katz, PhD, Georgetown University Medical Center, Washington, DC

Howard S. King, MD, Pediatric Office, Newton, MA

Alice Kitchen, LCSW, The Children's Mercy Hospital, Kansas City, MO

John Knight, MD, Children's Hospital, Boston, MA

Daniel P. Kohen, MD, University of Minnesota, Minneapolis, MN

Richard E. Kreipe, MD, Strong Memorial Hospital, Rochester, NY

John W. Kulig, MD, MPH, New England Medical Center, Boston, MA

Arthur Lavin, MD, St. Luke's Medical Office Center, Cleveland, OH

James Stuart Levi, MD, Mercer University School of Medicine, Macon, GA

Melvin D. Levine, MD, University of North Carolina at Chapel Hill, Chapel Hill, NC

Rolf Loeber, MD, West Psychiatric Institute and Clinics, Pittsburgh, PA

Chris Lonigan, PhD, Florida State University, Tallahassee, FL

Robert Mallard, MD, Greenshills Pediatric Associates, Nashville, TN

Arthur Maron, MD, FAAP, Saint Barnabas Medical Center, Livingston, NJ

Bruce J. Masek, PhD, Children's Hospital, Boston, MA

Patricia McGuire, MD, Health Source Pediatric Center, Cedar Rapids, IA

Ron McMillan, MD, American Psychiatric Association, Washington, DC

Carlo B. Melini, MD, FAAP, Robert Wood Johnson School of Medicine, Clinical Associates, Cooper Medical Center, Vineland, NJ

Gary Mesibov, MD, University of North Carolina, Chapel Hill, NC

Karen Miller, MD, Schneiders Children's Hospital, New Hyde Park, NY

James Moore, MD, Southdale Pediatric Associates, LTD, Edina, MD

David Moroney, MD, Old Harding Pediatrics, Nashville, TN

John Moses, MD, Duke University Medical Center, Durham, NC

John Nackaski, MD, University of Florida at Gainesville, Gainesville, FL

Philip R. Nader, MD, University of California - San Diego, LaJolla, CA

Richard Nelson, MD, The University of Iowa Hospitals and Clinics, Iowa, IA

Katherine Nitz, PhD, University of Maryland at Baltimore, Baltimore, MD

Robert B. Noll, PhD, Children's Hospital Medical Center, Cincinnati, OH

Audrey Hart Nora, MD, MPH, Maternal and Child Health Bureau, Rockville, MD

Thomas Ollendick, PhD, Virginia Polytechnic Institute and State University, Blacksburg, VA

Judith A. Owens-Stively, MD, MPH, Rhode Island Hospital, Providence, RI

John M. Pascoe, MD, MPH, University of Wisconsin Hospital, Madison, WI

David Pelcovitz, PhD, Cornell University Medical Center, Manhasset, NY

William E. Pelham, PhD, University of Pittsburgh Medical Center, Pittsburgh, PA

Lucille Perez, MD, National Medical Association, Rockville, MD

Ellen C. Perrin, MD, University of Massachusetts Medical Center, Worchester, MA

Theodore A. Petti, MD, MPH, Indiana University, Indianapolis, IN

Bruce W. Pfeffer, MD, Virginia Pediatric and Adolescent Center, Springfield, VA

Michael J. Philipp, PhD, DuPage County Health Department, Wheaton, IL

James Michael Pontious, MD, Enid Family Medicine Clinic, Enid, OK

Janice Prontnicki, MD, FAAP, Robert Wood Johnson Medical School, New Brunswick, NJ

David B. Pruitt, MD, University of Tennessee, Memphis, TN

William Rae, PhD, Scott and White Child And Adolescent Clinic, Temple, TX

Thomas H. Rand, MD, PhD, FAAP, Pediatric Associates, PA, Boise, ID

Leonard A Rappaport, MD, Children's Hospital, Boston, MA

Mark Reuben, MD, Reading Pediatrics, Wyomissing, PA

Anthony J. Richtsmeier, MD, Rush-Presbyterian-St. Luke's, Chicago, IL

William Risser, MD, PhD, UTMSH, Department of Pediatrics, Houston, TX

Dana S. Rubin, MD, Boston City Hospital, Boston, MA

David S. Rubovits, PhD, Mercy Hospital of Pittsburgh, Pittsburgh, PA

A. John Rush, MD, American Psychiatric Association, Dallas, TX

Sandra Russ, PhD, Case Western Reserve University, Cleveland, OH

Adrian Sandier, MD, University of North Carolina, Chapel Hill, NC

Richard M. Sarles, MD, University of Maryland at Baltimore, Baltimore, MD

Conway Saylor, PhD, Citadel, Charleston, SC

Barton Douglas Schmitt, MD, Children's Hospital, Denver, CO

Pamela A. Schmitz, Franklin Memorial Primary Health Care, Mobile, AL

Eric Schopler, MD, University of North Carolina, Chapel Hill, NC

Edward L. Schor, MD, Health Institute, New England Medical Center, Boston, MA

Manuel Schydlower, MD, Texas Tech. University, El Paso, TX

David Shaffer, MD, New York State Psychiatric Institute, New York, NY

Donald L. Shifrin, MD, Pediatric Associates, Bellevue, WA

William Shore, MD, Family and Community Medicine, University of California at San Francisco, San Francisco, CA

Terry Stancin, PhD, Metro Health Medical Center, Cleveland, OH

Ruth E. K. Stein, MD, Albert Einstein College of Medicine, Bronx, NY

Karl W. Stevenson, MD, FAPA, FAACAP, Psychiatric Associates of Durham, Durham, NC

J. Jordan Storlazzi, Jr., MD, PA, Pediatrics, Bloomington, DE

Raymond Sturner, MD, Duke University Medical Center, Durham, NC

Paula D. Sullivan, PhD, Indiana University School of Medicine, Riley Hospital for Children, Indianapolis, IN

Jack T. Swanson, MD, McFarland Clinic, Ames, IA

Ernest Walter Swihart, Jr., MD, South Lake Clinic/Pediatrics West, Minnetonka, MN

Arnold, L. Tanis, MD, FAAP, Pediatric Associates, P.A., Hollywood, CA

Kenneth J. Tarnowski, PhD, University of South Florida, Fort Meyers, FL

Raymond Tervo, MD, University of South Dakota School of Medicine-Pediatrics, Sioux Falls, SD

Mary Ann Timmis, PhD, Wayne State University, Detroit, MI

Richard Todd, MD, Washington University School of Medicine, St. Louis, MO

Deborah Tolchin, MD, University of Pediatrics, Bronx, NY

Elizabeth G. Triggs, MD, Green Hills Pediatrics Associates, Nashville, TN

John Trudeau, MD, Pediatric Services, Inc., Parma, OH

William B. Weil, Jr., MD, Michigan State University, East Lansing, MI

Mark Werner, MD, Vanderbilt, University of Nashville, TN

John S. Werry, MD, University of Auckland, Auckland, New Zealand

Mark Widome, MD, The Milton S. Hershey Medical Center, Hershey, PA

Serena Wieder, PhD, National Center for Clinical Infant Programs, Arlington, VA

David W. Willis, MD, Emanuel Hospital and Health Center, Portland, OR

Larry Wissow, MD, Johns Hopkins Hospital, Baltimore, MD

Gabriele Woloshin, MD, Cook County Hospital, Evanston, IL

Deborah Zarin, MD, American Psychiatric Association, Washington, DC

Phyllis C. Zee, MD, PhD, Northwestern University, Chicago, IL

Sara Kay Zirkle, MD, FAAP, Developmental and Behavioral Pediatrics, Richland, WA

Barry Zuckerman, MD, Boston City Hospital, Boston, MA

INDEX

INDEX

A

Abuse
  physical (995.5), 45
  sexual (995.5), 45
Academic skills, 69–75
  comorbid conditions, 75
  definitions and symptoms, 69
  developmental variation, 71
  differential diagnosis, 74
  disorder, 73–74
  epidemiology, 70
  etiology, 70
  presenting complaints, 69
  problem, 72
Acculturation (V62.4), 48
Acute health conditions (V61.49), 53
Acute stress disorder (308.3), 151
  diagnostic criteria for, 311
  in differential diagnosis, 198, 205
Addition of a sibling (V61.8), 47
Adjustment disorder, NOS (309.9), 313
Adjustment disorders (309.xx)
  as comorbid condition, 169, 266
  diagnostic criteria for, 312–313
  in differential diagnosis, 179, 198
Adjustment disorder with anxiety
    (309.24), diagnostic criteria
    for, 312
Adjustment disorder with depressed
    mood (309.0), 116, 158
  diagnostic criteria for, 312
  in differential diagnosis, 160
Adjustment disorder with disturbance of
    conduct (309.3), 124, 130
  diagnostic criteria for, 313
  in differential diagnosis, 131
Adjustment disorder with mixed anxiety
    and depressed mood (309.28),
    diagnostic criteria for, 312
Adjustment disorder with mixed
    disturbance of emotions and
    conduct (309.4), diagnostic
    criteria, 313
Adolescent gender identity disorder
    (302.85), 259
Adolescent occupational challenges
    (V62.2), 49
Adoption/institutional care (V61.29), 45
Adverse effect of work environment
    (V62.1), 49
Aggressive/oppositional behaviors, 119–126
  comorbid conditions, 126
  definitions and symptoms, 119
  developmental variation, 121–122
  differential diagnosis, 125
  disorder, 123–124
  epidemiology, 120
  etiology, 120
  presenting complaints, 119
  problem, 122–123

Aggressive/oppositional problem
    (V71.02), 122–123
  aggression, 123
  oppositionality, 122
Aggressive/oppositional variation
    (V65.49), 121–122
  aggression, 122
  oppositionality, 121
Alcohol abuse (305.00), 350. *See
    also* Substance use/abuse
Alcohol dependence (303.90), 349
Alcohol intoxication (303.00), 349
Amphetamine abuse (305.70), 349
Amphetamine dependence (304.40), 349
Anorexia nervosa (307.1), 231, 313
  as comorbid condition, 160, 164
  in differential diagnosis, 164, 225
Antisocial personality disorder (301.7),
    diagnostic criteria for, 313–314
Anxiety disorder, generalized (300.02), 149
  as comorbid condition, 67, 102, 110,
    131, 141, 160, 179, 188, 226,
    243, 260, 266
  diagnostic criteria for, 329–330
  in differential diagnosis, 100, 164, 198,
    205, 225
Anxiety disorder, NOS (300.00), 163
  as comorbid condition, 233
  diagnostic criteria for, 314–315
  in differential diagnosis, 198, 232
Anxiety disorder due to...(293.84),
    diagnostic criteria for, 314
Anxiety disorder due to a generalized
    medical condition (293.84),
    in differential diagnosis, 164
Anxiety problem (V40.2), 148
Anxiolytic. *See under* Sedative
Anxious symptoms, 145–152
  comorbid conditions, 152
  definitions and symptoms, 145–146
  developmental variation, 147
  differential diagnosis, 152
  disorder, 149–151
  epidemiology, 146
  etiology, 146
  presenting complaints, 145
  problem, 148
Anxious variation (V65.49), 147
Arousal conditions, partial, 189
Asperger's disorder (299.80), 282
  diagnostic criteria for, 315
Attachment relationship, as risk/
    protective factor, 34
Attachment relationship, challenges
    to (V61.20), 43
Attention-deficit/hyperactivity disorder
    (314.x), 93–94, 97–98, 107–108
  combined type (314.01), 98, 108, 315

as comorbid condition, 67, 75, 81, 89,
    118, 119, 131, 141, 160, 164,
    188, 226, 275
  in differential diagnosis, 74, 81, 152,
    160, 198, 205, 283
  NOS (314.9), 98, 108, 316
  predominantly hyperactive-impulsive
    (314.01), 97, 315
  predominantly inattentive (314.00),
    107, 316
Atypical behaviors, 267–289
  bizarre behaviors, 285–289
  repetitive behavioral patterns, 269–275
  social interaction behaviors, 277–284
Autistic disorder (299.00), 278, 281–282
  as comorbid condition, 67, 160, 243
  diagnostic criteria for, 316–317
  in differential diagnosis, 66, 74, 81, 89,
    100, 109, 164, 205, 213, 274
Avoidant personality disorder (301.82)
  as comorbid condition, 102
  diagnostic criteria for, 317
  in differential diagnosis, 100

B

Bed wetting. *See* Wetting problems
Behavioral clusters, 58. *See also*
    Childhood manifestations *and*
    individual clusters
  format of, 14
Bereavement (V62.82), 155
  as comorbid condition, 169
Binge eating, 221–226
  comorbid conditions, 226
  definitions and symptoms, 221–222
  developmental variation, 223
  differential diagnosis, 225
  disorder, 224
  epidemiology, 222
  presenting complaints, 221
  problem, 223
Bipolar disorders (296.xx), 286
  as comorbid condition, 169, 226
  in differential diagnosis, 232
Bipolar I disorder, most recent episode
    depressed (296.5x)
  as comorbid condition, 126
  diagnostic criteria for, 317
  in differential diagnosis, 125, 188
Bipolar I disorder, most recent episode
    hypomanic (296.40), diagnostic
    criteria for, 318
Bipolar I disorder, most recent episode
    manic (296.4x), diagnostic
    criteria for, 318
Bipolar I disorder, most recent episode
    mixed (296.6x), diagnostic criteria
    for, 319